THE TRUTH
ABOUT HEALING
What Big Medi$in Doesn't Want You To Know

"The Truth Shall Set You Free"

By
BERTRAM J. WONG

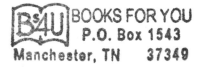

BOOKS FOR YOU
P.O. Box 1543
Manchester, TN   37349

The Truth About Healing
What Big Medi$in Doesn't Want You To Know

© COPYRIGHT 1998 BERTRAM J. WONG

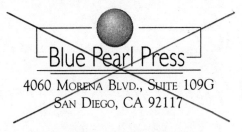

Blue Pearl Press

4060 MORENA BLVD., SUITE 109G
SAN DIEGO, CA 92117

TO ORDER ADDITIONAL COPIES OF THIS BOOK CALL:

931-728-5948

~~1-888-BOOKS-08~~

COVER DESIGN BY BERTRAM J. WONG
AND MICHAEL ANTHONY LYNCH

MANUFACTURED IN THE UNITED STATES OF AMERICA

ISBN: 1-891099-01-9

This book is not intended to replace the services of the health care industry. Its purpose is to provide the reader with facts from which he or she may develop a perspective of today's state of health and disease.

The use of masculine pronouns in this book will refer to persons of either gender.

Bertram Wong is available for lectures and seminars and can be booked through Blue Pearl Press at:

1-619-274-7614 OR 1-619-406-4006

DEDICATION

For my siblings of the human family:

Those who are caught up in the mainstream of misinformation flowing from the flute of the Pied Piper. May they soon develop the wisdom and strength to escape the rat race.

Those in the developing areas of our world who will inevitably be visited by the Piper. May they have the wisdom and strength to disregard his siren song.

Those who have the wisdom and courage to remain out of the mainstream of contemporary medical philosophy, who are willing to honor their god-given wisdom by governing their lives in accordance with the dictates of their own common sense and conscience.

Those health professionals who have had the courage to escape the mainstream of erroneous medical practice and have gone out on their own onto paths that promise more true health.

ACKNOWLEDGMENTS

I am indebted to the many researchers and writers who have had the courage of their convictions not only to believe in themselves but also to share the fruits of their labor with others. They have given me valuable insights and the courage to believe in my own observations and to write this love letter to my siblings of the human family.

My son Greg contributed much of the pre-publishing work of this book. Without his help and encouragement I might have succumbed to the difficulties and discouragements of amateur authorship.

PREFACE

You have just embarked on a wild ride into territory comparatively unexplored. If you've got the guts to stick with me, you're invited to participate in examining facets of life not often enough contemplated.

Why has this wild territory remained so unexplored, especially in this age of virtually unlimited communication? Well, it's not completely unexplored. Free-thinking, open-minded men and women have tried to show us this beautiful realm of nature but have been no match for the moneyed entities who have axes to grind and whose interests would not be served by our knowledge of good and evil.

Let us leave the metaphoric scene and get down to straight talk. You may regard this as a letter from me to you. Though I offer very valid health information, that will be my secondary and incidental purpose only. Primarily I will attempt to dissuade you from the mainstream of current medical philosophy onto a path which promises more health and less disease and suffering — a lot more and a lot less. This superior approach has been impugned, maligned, and all but obscured by modern commercial interests.

After suffering and laboring through the crucible of disease, earning a degree in the College of Hard Knocks, poring over numerous books and articles by health experts of all stripes, distinguishing to the best of my ability between the intelligent and the naive, the sincere and those excessively profit-oriented, the thinker and the parrot, I have written here the essence of my conclusions on the subject.

Can 40 million Frenchmen be wrong? Can 260 million Americans be wrong? Can 100 U.S. Senators be wrong? Can 435 U.S. Representatives be wrong? Is our government running smoothly, free of budgetary deficits and debt? Can millions of American doctors be wrong? Is our quality of life improving? Is our health improving? Are we needing fewer hospitals now? Are the rates of arthritis and cancer mitigating?

It has been said that the majority are always wrong. That depends. If just being good enough is good enough for us, then I guess the majority are pretty close to being right most of the time. But if we are to strive for the best possible life, to be uncommon, to be somebody rather than anybody, then we had better seek our answers not from the pied pipers and lemmings of society but from some Good Shepherd, and perhaps also be good shepherds ourselves.

"Rather than love, than money, than fame, give me truth."

— Henry David Thoreau

I am not a writer in search of grist for his craft. A message cries out to be shared with you, and I have chosen to write my letter in the form of *The Truth About Healing, What Big Medi$in Doesn't Want You To Know.*

As you contemplate the validity of my reasoning and compare the opposing forces of truth and falsehood, among your key considerations might be: "Who has an axe to grind?" and "Am I happy with the work of the present medical powers-that-be?" If you say you're happy, you're dismissed. I can't help you. But I'll try to visit you in the nursing home in between my tennis matches.

If you have any respect at all for your own mind and spirit, any reverence for your Creator, any regard for the uniqueness of your thinking processes, then in the name of your beingness and aliveness, don't waste them. Be willing to think for yourself and value the products of your wondrous mind. Refrain from summarily accepting the conventional wisdoms of the "experts" and "authorities" simply because they are axioms and dogmas. Especially objectionable is living one's life in accordance with these bromides even when they have clearly shown they don't work, just because everyone else seems to believe them.

Reject what doesn't work and espouse what does. Be your own authority, as long as you don't try to be everyone else's. Then you can keep a confident hand on the reins of your life and perhaps help our children to do the same.

"So long as a man thinketh for himself he is free."
— Ralph Waldo Emerson

"...thou shalt see through thine own eyes and not through the eyes of others, and shalt know of thine own knowledge and not of the knowledge of thy neighbors."
— Baha'Ulah

The Truth About Healing, What Big Medi$in Doesn't Want You To Know is not in accord with orthodox medicine, which, by the way, has very little to do with health except in a negative sense. Not only is it not in keeping with that revered science; more than that I will undertake to debunk almost all the major tenets of a monstrous industry which purports to keep us well but in reality has kept its trusting customers in bondage by hoodwinking them into believing it is omniscient and staffed by god-men. I have seen and suffered too much and too long to sit idly by and watch you and our people further abused and exploited mercilessly.

"Silence isn't always golden; sometimes it is yellow."
— Author unknown

"Lord, give me... the strength to change the things I can."
— Epictetus

Yes, this book is iconoclastic, but not for the sake of being contrary. After all, mere tradition doesn't necessarily make for truth. Please read with a thoughtful mind and a questing spirit and in the end decide for yourself whether my theses are worthy of further contemplation.

I am not asking you to agree with me any more than I want you to go along with the so-called authorities. I will share with you knowledge, opinions if you prefer, wrested from decades of a tough curriculum in the College of Hard

Knocks. My instructors were Mother Nature and numerous Doctors of Medicine, whom I shall sometimes refer to as M.D.s. Mother has taught me very well in the various aspects of life: physical, mental, and spiritual. I have also garnered valuable knowledge from the medical industry but not what they intended to teach me and you. Most of their information I consider to be incorrect; fallacious or collusive may be a more accurate and candid description. The late Will Rogers, beloved American humorist, was not far wrong when he said, "A lot of folks knows a lot of things that ain't so." Isn't it ironical that the word "doctor" is translated from the Greek word that means "teacher?"

Nobody on this planet abhors waste any more than I do. I suffer extreme discomfort in the idea that all my interesting thoughts, all my valued knowledge eked out over my long lifetime, should vanish and count for utter naught when my lights are finally switched off. To prevent such a tragedy is one of the purposes of this endeavor.

Personally counting for something is another purpose. It is often said that a measure of a person's worth is what he contributes to his world. I hope I and my gift will count for something. When my account is finally balanced and closed, will I have given my world more than I have received?

Another purpose is self preservation, the strongest instinct in man. I do not relish the prospects of my footprints' being washed away by the first high tide. I want to be remembered favorably. I want my children to know that their Dad left something of value behind for their generation, to know me and my soul. In other words I want to be loved, even when I'm gone. Thereby I will live on.

"The great use of life is to spend it for something that outlasts it."

— William James

As you will gather when you read on, my life has been fraught with frustrations and failures. This is not false modesty. I am being very candid with you. My failures are a very essential part of my message to you. If I am to help you I cannot defer to my pride. I will try to show you how you can enhance your chances of avoiding the suffering I have experienced. What is this they say about studying the past in order not to repeat mistakes? So perhaps you understand that for me this difficult project is a first and last hurrah. Successful or not, it is my effort to salvage a modicum of worthiness. Now I can feel much better about myself as I leave this realm knowing that I have tried to make this a better world.

Perhaps my strongest reason for this book is my love and appreciation of God and my love for His precious children. I cannot rest while my brothers and sisters continue to rely on a system that clearly has drained them of their health and wealth and promises to drain even more, whatever little of them is left. In the face of this terrible abuse the world is crying out for a healing, and I'm trying to help.

I have stood before a mirror and said to myself, "Hey, man, perhaps you had better rethink your theses. If five billion people disagree with you they may have good reason to." But I have not been able to reconcile with the huge majority. If my theses are correct and therefore beneficial, then all the more should they be promulgated lest the concepts fail to see the light of day for another untenable eon.

In the face of an intolerable impasse, a seemingly hopeless plight, somebody must venture outward, explore new possibilities, and report his findings to his fellows for evaluation. If new knowledge emerges perhaps the hopelessness and impasse will mitigate and mankind will be able to reclaim its God-given heritage. Such an impasse is now upon us. But you already know this.

Is one to be considered a quixotic fool who dares to make brazen pronouncements in head-on contradiction of a sophisticated multi-billion dollar science purported to be the ultimate in loving care? Is he a buffoon who chooses certain ridicule in exchange for a perceived possibility that millions of his human siblings will be delivered from the intolerable impasse and walk again on the sunny side of the street? If so, so be it. A buffoon is born every day. But if you don't mind, I prefer to be called eccentric, because being out-of-center sometimes affords one a better view not shared by those immobilized by the crowd's restricting their every move.

I tried for many years to write this book, intending it to be of substance and dignity, a product of thorough research and documentation. But having a busy life to live I did not measure up to the task. And so my endeavor remained in limbo for much of the time. At one point I made a clean break of it and tossed out all the volumes of notes and articles I had accumulated. But my conscience would not let go, because the agents of greed, deceit, and suffering would not let go. And so I could not turn my back on my responsibility.

"Remorse is regret that one waited so long to do it."
— H. L. Menken

"Regret for time wasted can become a power for good in the time that remains, if we will only stop the waste and the idle useless regretting."
— Arthur Brisbane

Here are the fruits of my soul. They are not excerpted from sophisticated tomes of technical literature. Most of them come from my years of suffering, study, and learning, including practical articles and books by persons much less "educated" than the professionals of Big Medi$in. Clearly this is not a textbook for scientists and professors. It is a love offering to you my beloved.

"What is a man born for but to be a reformer, a remaker of what has been made, a denouncer of lies, a restorer of truth and good?"
— Ralph Waldo Emerson

"Every man is guilty of all the good he didn't do."
— Voltaire

First I will tell you the story of my long years of puzzling misery due to an immobilizing condition of mind and body. Then I hope you will be outraged when you learn how ironically I obtained a good measure of dramatic relief almost overnight from my years of suffering which had been totally unnecessary but obviously nurtured as a cash cow. The episode in which I was freed from my misery was the birth of my enlightenment in the machinations of Big Medi$in. The powerful impression made on my psyche by what I had learned of the modus operandi of the ostensible caretakers of our health inspired me to take a keen interest in what a beautiful and marvelous gift God has given us, what health really is, how it is obtained and maintained, who is killing us, and why and how they are doing it. What I learned is not taught in medical school and not what is foisted on us laymen by our medical heroes. Far from it. And what I learned from others has been solidly confirmed by my own experience.

Am I downright presumptuous when I dare contradict the thousands of volumes of sophisticated scientific literature within the hallowed halls of prestigious institutions of higher learning? Amen. But even a mouse may look at an emperor, and this time the emperor again has no clothes.

Following the story of my education I will share with you what I have learned about your wondrous body which is so lovingly nurtured by Mother Nature. I refer to it as Mother's Marvelous Machine. Here the discussion will center more on you. I want you to be involved. And here especially I want you to exercise your personal sovereignty in contemplating the unusual, though logical, explanations.

You will eventually notice that I care comparatively little about specific symptoms, holding firmly to the concept that symptoms are merely symptoms. However, following the chapter on Mother's Marvelous Machine I will discuss several popular ones. But you will also gather from the discussions that my underlying purpose will be to point out the oneness of your entire body and mind, the mutual integrity of all their parts, and the relative insignificance of symptoms.

Then will come the chapter on Big Medi$in, perhaps the most important thrust of the book. It could be the most beneficial, depending on the degree of your receptivity to the facts. It will be devoted mostly to my evaluation of orthodox medicine as it is committed in the U.S. of A. Any practice must have its practitioners and so the American M.D. will have his share of attention. Alternative disciplines of the healing arts also will be examined.

Discussing a problem without trying to provide a solution leaves the job half-done, and so in conclusion I will offer you my version of what health is and how it can be obtained and maintained.

Should you feel the need to dispute any of my commentaries, be my guest. But as the late Jimmy Durante said, "Include me out." Follow your own star. My offerings are my own and hold no technical authority. They are the fruits of that venerable institution of learning which instead of paper credit awards its students solid knowledge of life, but only if they seek it with a receptive and questing mind and spirit.

"Ye shall know the truth and the truth shall set you free."
— The Holy Bible

Above all I hope to have stimulated your thinking and have a hand in your gaining new concepts to explore.

TABLE OF CONTENTS

INTRODUCTION

As you go through this amazing book, I am certain you will feel as I did that Bertram Wong is having a conversation with no one but you. His direct personal approach is responsible for this intimate feeling, just as his humor is a welcome boon to a very serious subject. The personalization and the humor underscore his poignant messages.

Mr. Wong pulls no punches as he relates his own progression of good-health concepts. His honesty is refreshing, and his intuition will make you wonder how he knows about events that have occurred in *your* life, events that surely every one of us must have experienced. You will smite your forehead again and again, and say, "Yep! That's me!"

To those of us who have struggled over the years to tell many of the same stories, Wong's message is not new. But he tells it in a most compelling way. When you are young, it's hard to know what it is like to be old. When you are well, it's hard to know what it is like to be sick. Wong gives his readers a clear image of these states, even for those for whom these messages may now seem far removed from reality. So, please: pay attention!

Many of the quotes he uses — well-known, for the most part — will not only take on new meaning, but will help you to remember what he is teaching.

Although the title of the book suggests a certain negativity (and, yes, Wong does strike against Big Medi$in), the chapters are actually filled with hope!

Wong's impassioned pleas for you to change your ways are speckled with advice of precisely how to do this. The book is a tour de force — an amazing compilation of lifestyle facets which, if followed, can keep us all in good health.

Betty Kamen, Ph.D.

CHAPTER ONE

COLLEGE OF HARD KNOCKS

"I have but one lamp by which my feet are guided and that is the lamp of experience,"
—Patrick Henry, 1779

I am one of the world's greatest underachievers. I say this not to reflect favorably on my native abilities or to berate myself for being lazy. For native ability by definition is not earned and therefore not a credit, just a windfall. In fact, for many years, sensing my potential abilities, I was very ashamed of my failure to accomplish anything of substance, like getting enough "B"s and "C"s in school, even though I was often called a genius. Officially my IQ is 153, which qualifies me for membership in MENSA, an international organization of the top 2% of intellectuals worldwide. That's really not too much to scream about, but astronomical alongside my "D"s and "F"s. As for my being lazy, you will eventually understand and hopefully have a little more compassion, as I have, for persons accused of being lazy. I will be telling you of numerous shortfalls in achievement relative to my inherent capabilities. Most of my life has been a story of gross under achievement and failures. Here I will try to show you how terribly a life can be shortchanged and wasted by poor inner health. But eventually the major reason for my woes will be discovered and will be a major factor in my writing this book.

1

Until my mid-thirties my life was one of profound frustration. At an early age I became acutely aware of some indefinable condition which was like a ball and chain not only around my ankle but also around my mind. I could feel it all too well but could not describe it even to myself, much less do anything to free myself from it.

Eventually I got to see the monster's face but not until I was in my forties, after many long agonizing years of confusion and much too late to start building a foundation for my life. But we're getting ahead of the story. When you eventually meet the monster I will want you to know him very well, because he is one of the star characters in the plot and may very well be a significant character in the plot of your life. I will also want you to know a few other monsters whose ilk certainly do play a part in all of our lives.

This narrative is not meant to be a fun story. It is what I consider a practical way of laying the groundwork for your understanding of what I will discuss with you a bit later on.

So let's go 'way back and start our journey at the beginning. My memory goes back to age two, in the little town of Kapaa on the island of Kauai in the Hawaiian chain. That's when my long years of troubles began, except that I did not then recognize them as troubles, for they were pleasurable. But, as the saying goes, nothing is free, and imprudence, willful or in ignorance, must some day be paid for.

For about two years, probably every day, I stuffed concentrated sweet carbohydrates into my tender little physiology. Unfortunately these carbos were not very complex. The only complexity about them was that I could never decide which I liked best.

Undoubtedly, with apologies to my siblings and my next-door cousins, I was my grandfather's favorite child,

2

even though he lived in the home of these cousins and their parents. As I recall, he took me for a walk around town just about every day and always bought me one, two, or all three of my favorite goodies: Cracker Jack, "red soda water," and those sugar-soaked coconut balls dyed a brilliant red on the outside.

When Grandpa wasn't indulging my hedonistic penchant for sugar, which probably he himself was responsible for developing, I sometimes sojourned to the little store operated by my aunt and uncle immediately in front of our home on the same property. For there on a couple of old benches outside the front wall of the store I could almost always find a half-dozen old men among whom there was always at least one who was more than willing to satisfy my craving for the sweet stuff. But those goodies were no more free than a free lunch. I always had to suffer the indignity of good-natured teasing, the kind that old men usually enjoy at the expense of helpless little boys. Their favorite was to bring out their sharp pocket knives and threaten to cut off my little peanut. Now, out of six-or-so old men with nothing else to do one could almost always find at least one with little enough sense and consideration to carry out his act with too much realism, and I don't mind telling you those were scary times. And these episodes were what kept me from meandering in that direction much more often. Nevertheless, no risk, no sweets, and so I often enough braved the dreaded surgery in favor of my insatiable addiction to life's greatest pleasures.

Those store treats were not the only objects of my cravings. At home one of my favorites was "sugar bread." A bakery was almost next-door to our home, and the hot, fresh aromatic bread we often got intensified my addiction. A thick hand-cut slice of the fragrant stuff was plastered with yummy butter and then topped with a layer of beautiful white sugar which emitted the prettiest sound when chewed into. You just don't know what good is.

Other junk foods also accommodated my appetite those young days and earned me the name Fat among my playmates. I am certain I consumed much more sugar and starches than most children my age or any age.

Then there was rice — beautiful, slightly sweet, hot white rice. I ate much more of it than other children, and this preference was encouraged by my grandfather. He believed, probably along with other Chinese sages of old, that the child who ate more rice relative to the other goodies on the table showed frugality and therefore character and a sense of responsibility. "This is a good boy. He's not spoiled."

I lost some of my baby teeth very early. Photographs show me without my front teeth when I was three or four. I recall having an excruciatingly painful boil on my leg just before my fourth birthday. I also recall having a snotty nose.

About that time we moved to the town of Kilauea on the same island, where my father was bookkeeper for a large sugar plantation. The move was probably very fortunate for me in that my intake of sugar was considerably curtailed, as my grandfather remained in the other town. But I still ate sugar bread and all the sweets I could stuff into my mouth. I learned from my father the fine art of eating an avocado; namely, filling the seed cavity with gleaming white sugar and then you know what. Try it some time. Or mash the avocado with sugar and almond extract and spread it as thick as you can on a slice of fresh bread. What am I saying!

I don't recall very much about the state of my health the two-years-or-so we lived in Kilauea, but I do remember my runny nose.

My mother was a school teacher and started me in first grade when I was five. The "ABC"s were a breeze and I kept wondering why we had to keep studying the same old stuff over and over again.

After two years in Kilauea we moved to Wahiawa on the island of Oahu, on which Honolulu, the capital city of Hawaii, is situated. Young school teachers were moved around quite a bit those days. My father took a position as bookkeeper at Schofield Barracks, then America's largest military outpost with 20,000 men. It was about then that I began to really feel sub-par physically. I was six. Saturday mornings were clean-house time, and we children, five of us, were assigned chores. It was a strange phenomenon, but invariably I felt extremely weak and tired when trying to do my share of the housework, even after a heavy breakfast. Guilt feelings were very much in the forefront of my consciousness, as I couldn't help surmising that I lacked esprit de corps and that as a result my mind failed to drum up the enthusiasm to inspire my body to scrub the walls or clean the windows. Of course I didn't think in these words, but I didn't need words to feel the way I did. How was I to know then that it was not laziness but that there was a very valid explanation for that kind of reaction on my part? And how was I to know then that I was weak and tired not in spite of a heavy breakfast but because of it? We will explore those ramifications of physiology a bit later.

I woke up ravenously hungry every morning and ate a much heavier breakfast than my parents ever knew about. As a school teacher my mother didn't have the luxury of time to supervise our eating. After placing our food on the table she hurried out of the kitchen to prepare for her day's responsibilities. And that was when we did our thing. It was a daily routine for me to consume half of my three sisters', and sometimes my brother's, oatmeal. As soon as Mother was out of the kitchen several bowls would be slid across the table to me, or sometimes they would be lifted and poured out of. ("You should never end a sentence with a preposition." Poppycock.) Of course I would always add more sugar to the new supply, and sometimes strawberry jam. It was a symbiotic arrangement. My siblings got away with eating less of the vile stuff and I got to eat more of the sweet stuff. Two conditions inspired my great intake of food: my rabid appetite and a seemingly innate antipathy for waste. At times when I thought I had arrived at the limits of my capacity and refused to accept any more of the surplus, all my sisters had to do to change my mind was to head for the sink drain with their bowls. I was often called Garbage Can. I'm still a packrat today.

It was this sudden heavy intake of sugar on a hungry stomach that did me in, as will be elaborated on when we discuss the workings of our bodies.

After three years in Wahiawa we moved back to Honolulu, where I had been born in 1919. I still had a perpetual runny nose and many spells of weakness. I was now in the fourth grade and having a difficult time in school. I got my classroom work done well enough, despite frequent dozing, but could not do the homework worth a hoot. When our teacher Miss Morita asked me about my not doing my assignments I could never give her an answer that was anywhere near sensible or logical, and that was because I simply did not know. I did not realize that I lacked the mental energy to cope with even a few minutes of mental work. At best it was a confounding situation. I was confused.

Learning the lessons in the classroom was no big problem, even though I often fell asleep. If grades throughout my scholastic career had been based on test results alone, I would have made the honor roll most of the time. Unfortunately homework assignments counted for a lot, and so I was a poor student. Apparently I had a good steering system but not enough fuel to go anywhere.

One afternoon after school Miss Morita took me with her to the University of Hawaii, where I was seated at a little table in front of a huge audience in a huge auditorium. On the other side of the table was an elderly gentleman, whom I now presume to have been a psychology professor of some kind, who questioned me for what seemed to be about two hours, after which members of the audience questioned me. The staff at the University concluded that I had an extraordinarily capable mind but were probably as unable as Miss Morita and my mother to explain my unusual demeanor as a student. It was then that I first learned the word genius. This mystery was to persist and puzzle all of my teachers until I finally dropped out of college in my sophomore year.

Every single year from fourth grade on through high school, sometimes several times a year, one, two, or three teachers would keep me between classes or after school and the conversation would go very much like this:

"Bert, I don't understand you. You seem to handle the work so easily and you seem to understand everything I teach the class, even though you're asleep half the time. But why is it you don't do your homework, even on important projects? Why don't you care about your responsibilities?"

"I do care, Miss Falk." (Miss Signi Falk was one of my teachers in my high school sophomore year. I respected

7

and loved her dearly and was extremely sorry to be letting her down.)

"You do? It certainly doesn't seem that you do."

"I do care, and I try to do my work. But I can't."

"What do you mean, you can't? I know better. This work is easy for you. Tell me why you can't do your homework. Do you have too much other work to do at home?"

"No."

"Then why, Bert, why? You're not cooperating with me. You should be able to give me some kind of answer and then maybe we can go on from there and help you get your work done. Can you try to explain to me why you can't do your work?"

"Sorry, Miss Falk. I can't."

"You can't do the work or you can't explain?"

"I can't do the work and I don't know why."

"Bert, do you realize I'm trying to help you? It hurts me to see a bright boy like you not making use of his brains."

"Yes, Miss Falk, I appreciate that you're trying to help me. In fact you're my favorite teacher. But I guess there's something crazy in my head."

"No, Bert, you're not crazy. Listen. I'm going to keep trying to figure you out. In the meantime you try your best, okay?"

"Okay. I'll try."

"I know you'll try. For me, okay?" Then Miss Signi Falk placed both her hands on my shoulders, looked at me tenderly, and kissed me on the cheek. Then and there I wished I were about 28 years old.

Well, like all my teachers before and after her, Miss Falk could do nothing for me, the terrible enigma. What hurt me a lot was that none of them knew how helpless I felt inside and how much I wished I could figure myself out and take my rightful place on the honor roll alongside some of those dummies who weren't as smart as I was. My big goal every term was to not get an "F" and not too many "D"s, and I can't say I was eminently successful in that endeavor. In the five six-term years I attended that school, thirty terms in all, I never made the honor roll, let alone come near making it. But hold on now. I did receive the Honor Pin once, for one six-week term, and that entitled me to be called an Honor Man. To earn the Pin one had to have all his grades a "B" or better and must not have violated any regulation. This honor was not the same as making the honor roll, which required all grades to be "A"s. So you can see it was no big deal, a sort of consolation prize, or an honorable mention in a contest. But hey, let's not belittle my big deal, okay? It was a momentous achievement not only for me but for quite a few of my teachers as well. "Atta boy, Bert! (Some of them called me Bertram.) I told you you could do it!"

I wore that blasted Honor Pin all of one day. That very evening I was arraigned by the Student Senate and found guilty of violating some stupid regulation. Ironically that was one of my very few official violations in all my five years there. But no matter. I had to give up the Pin anyway, right there on the spot. That one day, though not a full 24 hours, turned out to be the crowning glory of my illustrious scholastic career. I wrote an English composition entitled "King For a Day," and Miss Falk gave me an "A+" for it, saying she loved it. But perhaps she was just trying to help me maintain the momentum that earned me the fluke award. Be that as it may; that was that. I didn't want that damned Pin anyway.

A year before that, one day when I was a ninth-grader in plane geometry class, the entire class with the exception of me were in unanimous accord on a problem. I expressed my opinion and was roundly booed. "Sit down, Bert. You're off the beam!" We went 'round and 'round for quite a while, with some of us flailing at the blackboard. Finally our teacher Mr. Ray Stewart said, "Sorry, class, but Bert is right." Then he took over the blackboard and convinced everybody else, officially anyway, of the correct approach to the problem. Later in the semester we, the class versus me, had another altercation, similar to the previous one. Similar argument prevailed. In due time Mr. Stewart said, "Sorry, Bert, but this time I'll have to say I'm siding with the class."

"Okay. Why?"

So Mr. Stewart went to the blackboard with his theoretical explanation. Aha! I spotted the flaw in his theorizing, jumped up, and pointed it out to him and the class. He looked at it intently for a long time and finally said, "Class, I'm afraid Bert is right again, and we're all wrong, including myself."

From then on, for the remainder of my high school years, Mr. Stewart seemed to exude profound respect for me at our every contact. As we were in a boarding school, that was often.

In my senior year four of us had a neat little racket going. My buddy and I with our respective girl friends often sneaked behind the Teachers' Parlor after dinner to do some innocent smooching between the building and the tall hibiscus hedge. One evening whom should we see there but Ray Stewart and Bernardine Downey, a pretty young teacher at our school, doing exactly what we were planning to do. We looked at each other a fleeting moment and then in mutual respect and understanding went about our own

10

businesses. I have no compunction about telling on Ray, because he and Bernardine eventually got married and presumably lived happily ever after. Moreover, I could now call him on a first-name basis, only in private of course, because we now had more in common. The next morning Ray saw me at the far end of a corridor and walked over to me. He put his arm around my shoulder and gave me a heartfelt hug. "Bert, you're my real buddy!"

Incidentally, this little interlude of my high school days had a delayed ending, an ignominious one, about 38 years later. When my wife and I visited Molokai, one of the outer Hawaiian islands, I decided to look up Mary, my former smooching partner. Guess what. You won't believe this, but much to my chagrin and my wife's delight Mary didn't remember me! (!!??) C'mon now! How in the world...? I guess our innocent smooching was too innocent. Or perhaps Mary was already senile. Moreover, in her middle fifties she wasn't the tender cherubic beauty she was at sixteen anyway. But whatever, there was another case of under achievement! Didn't I do anything right?

All my life I've had trouble staying awake in any kind of class. Even at fascinating seminars for which I pay good money I fall asleep. I still sleep in church every Sunday. In grade school I slept so much in class that I deservedly earned the name Lullaby. And that was no one-time or short-term nickname; that was my name. In high school my Latin teacher had our principal send me to the school doctor downtown to find out what was wrong with me. The doctor didn't know, of course, because doctors didn't know, still don't know, or don't want to know, much about what was bothering me then as well as in all the years before that. At the University as a sophomore I was in Chemistry 101, because I had flunked that course the year before. With

11

"W" the initial of my last name my seat was far back in the lecture auditorium. One afternoon I was shocked awake by a booming voice in an accusatory tone from down front. "Mr. Wong, if you stayed home at night instead of carousing around town you wouldn't have to sleep in class!" And of course there was the inevitable laughter. The hell of it was that I never was much of a carouser those days, being sick in mind and body. But I was somewhat accustomed to this kind of embarrassment, so it was okay. It had to be okay, because there wasn't a thing I could do about it.

On the night of our high school graduation ceremony our principal Mr. Anderson, a large man with reddish bushy eyebrows and characteristically reticent and intimidating, feigned a punch to my stomach and said, "Bert, you ol' bean!" I was surprised when he put his arm around my shoulder and gave me an expressive squeeze, something I had never seen him do to anyone. When he started to speak in hushed tones to my mother, I moseyed away to afford them privacy to speak freely, but not far enough to be out of earshot. I slipped behind the big man and eavesdropped. He told my mother that among the several thousand high school graduates in Hawaii that year I had placed second in the college aptitude tests. My first cousin Donna came in first. He also said that he had never had a student who so often thought differently from everyone else but who seemed always to have good basis for his opinion, also saying he liked the way I always thought for myself and was not excessively influenced by what others said.

Understandably I had not been recommended for college work and had not been accepted for matriculation that fall. In fact I had graduated only by the skin of my teeth, and I am certain Miss Taylor was only being charitable. In a way that was perfectly okay with me, because

I wasn't particularly eager to continue fighting the books anyway. But on the other hand my dear mother was keenly disappointed about it, and so on balance I decided to try for a reversal of the University's attitude toward me. I think these days they call that an attitude adjustment. I made two impassioned visits that summer to the Director of Admissions and in August miraculously convinced him to let me enroll for the coming term. His acquiescence was understandably reluctant and was based on my high rating on the tests. But I did not get away without being subjected to an intense lecture on what was to be expected of me as a student. I said, "Dr. Livesay, I appreciate this very much and will do my best to justify your faith in me."

"I know you will, Mr. Wong. Good luck to you."

I took Dr. Livesay's admonishments very seriously and that fall did fairly well, getting a 2.3 grade point average for the first semester. The second semester I think I got a 1.9, still not too bad for me, considering. Then came a 1.7 for the first semester of my sophomore year, and when I could stand no more of fighting the books, the assignments, and myself, I finally dropped out. I did not actually drop out; I simply ran out of fuel and my engine just couldn't squeeze out another mile. Period. Kaput. Oh, where was that proverbial bowl of cherries?

Let me get ahead of my story a spell and tell you about my later scholastic activities, just so we can dispense with that nasty subject once and for all. About twenty years later, having partially solved my health problems, I took night courses at the University to satisfy certain requirements of my work at the Pearl Harbor Naval Shipyard. These courses were in engineering, and I'm proud to tell you that, as I recall, I got nothing but "A"s and "B"s. One of the "A"s was in Applications of Calculus, no less.

13

Not too bad for an erstwhile dummy, eh? With the vast improvement in my health, my mind and emotions were in far better condition than in the bad old days. I must admit, however, to having thrown Dr. Linus Paulings's heavy-reading chemistry textbook through my living room window when I could tolerate no more of the agony. But I did get an "A" for that course. I eventually ended up with 118 college credits but never a degree. For one thing, I never needed one, and for another, those credits were in split majors and so I was not as close to a sheepskin as it would appear. So, so much for formal academics.

I have discussed the ball and chain around my mind and later I will tell you how I gained partial freedom from them. But in the physical realm my problems were no less vexing. In fact they were taken much more seriously by an immature youngster who placed more value on physical aspects. I recall with deep remorse how my sick mind and body hampered me in every sports activity in which I participated. This is not to imply that my sports were all that suffered. I felt awful all the time.

When I was about nine, I think it was a flea bite that started a sore on my leg. That bothersome sore festered seemingly forever, but actually only about two years. I don't know how much zinc ointment, gauze, and adhesive plaster I used. Band-Aid had not yet been conceived. I still have a very visible reminder of that sore today.

Though I was puzzled and frustrated by the persistence of that sore then, I understand it very well now and in fact am grateful for its having served its purpose. Odd that I should take this attitude, but if you don't read me now, you will when we discuss this important aspect in Mother's Marvelous Machine.

I could tell you of numerous physical, mental, and emotional unpleasantries that incessantly sprang from my mysteriously degenerated body. But that's a glum subject, and enough is enough.

Beginning my eighth-grade year I changed schools. The new one was a boarding school very close to my home in Honolulu. So understandably almost all of the students came from out-of-town, a few from country towns on Oahu, the same island, but most from plantation towns on the outlying islands. It was extraordinarily advantageous for those country natives, as it served as a sheltered introduction to the urbane life of a big city. But for me it was a five-year black hole in my young life. About ninety percent of the 150-or-so boys were of Japanese ancestry and from country towns where most of the residents were also Japanese. In fact some of them held dual citizenships, American and Japanese. Perhaps you are beginning to see why I had it so tough there, being of Chinese ancestry and fresh from a so-called English Standard school, where no student was enrolled unless he spoke very good English. For five long years I heard the Japanese language spoken day and night. And often that included the word "Shinajin," which literally meant a Chinese person, but to some of the boys, given the social context in which it was spoken, it undoubtedly connotatively meant a Chinaman. I'm not saying they were all racists. Individually they probably averaged out pretty well, if you make allowances for their narrowly racial beginnings. But collectively they were ethnically oriented and obviously thoroughly happy to be living among their own kind.

By the way, the school was coeducational, with fewer than a hundred girls of a more balanced racial mix. I liked the girls better. I still do.

15

The student body was divided into six clubs for the purpose of intramural competition of all kinds, especially sports, with even distribution of students from the various class levels. This arrangement was obviously much better than pitting eighth-graders against seniors. At the start of every sports season each club elected a captain from its membership to run the team for that season's competition. The only thing wrong with that otherwise good system was that no faculty supervision was provided, and so, given the ethnic loyalty of those country boys, poor Bertram never got to participate in any sports competition until his senior year, and then it was only in one sport. All through those years, even as a senior, I sat on the bench while eighth- and ninth-graders competed for our club. I was a good athlete and everybody knew it, because I was out on the athletic field as much as anyone. I had the capability to play on the varsity baseball team, but that too was a closed shop. The coach was of Japanese descent also and had formerly played and coached in Japan. In all those five years I never saw a notice soliciting a turnout from the student body at large. I used to punt a football over seventy yards consistently but never got to do it in competition. School coach Mr. Al Miller said I was a phenomenon and should be kicking for a professional team, even though I weighed only 120 pounds. Teacher Mr. Roger Davis insisted that I should kick for the University of Hawaii Rainbows after graduation from high school and also turn out for the hurdles in track. So you can understand that I was resentful and bitter about having been so bottled up.

I may as well finish talking about kicking a football. A fellow named Henry "Mongoose" Leandro was famous all over Honolulu for his punting ability and kicking the football 80 yards, though I have no way of knowing whether he did. One day I saw him kicking the ball around with some of his friends. Though I had always been some sort of "shrinking violet," I somehow drummed up the temerity to join this group of more matured athletes with whom I was not the least acquainted. Of course I made sure I would kick from where Mongoose was kicking. I stood there among them for a while until a friendly one said, "'Ey, kid, you like kick?" I said okay and he tossed me the ball. I boomed one over the heads of the fellows at the other end. Nobody said a word, probably thinking it was a fluke, but of course I knew they were impressed. The ball rotated among us for a while, and when I had kicked about three times one of them said, "'Ey, Canoe, (Mongoose was known as Canoe among his closer friends.) da kid kick mo' fa' den you." Leandro, usually a reticent fellow, mumbled, "Today my off-day."

Time passed. It so turned out that about eleven years later Mr. Leandro became my tenant by way of my real estate broker. I went to the house to get acquainted with my new tenant. When my knock on the door was answered I said, "Hello. I'm your landlord."

Immediately Mr. Leandro replied with, "Yeah, I know you. You used to hang around Makiki Park."

The funny thing about that was that I never did hang around Makiki Park, mainly because I had been in boarding school and we had classes on Saturdays. The only time I ever did anything in Makiki Park was when I kicked the football with Mongoose Leandro and his friends. So the famous punter obviously remembered that day — and me.

But let's get back to my high school days — not that they are a pleasant memory. There were a few boys of ethnic origins other than Japanese who got to participate in intramural competition. A few even sat on the bench of the varsity basketball team. But the coach here was Mr. Al Miller of Ohio, and that made a difference. So what does this say about me and my complaints? Yes, it was partly my own fault, in fact largely so. Yes, those Japanese boys were clannish, but given my abilities, with a normal personality I should have been able to take my rightful place in that social environment. But my personality was not normal, not even near normal. I had always been doggedly independent, resentful, even defiant, since childhood. I never asked for an allowance, never asked for food, never asked for anything, despite my abnormally excessive appetite. I did have the guts, however, to serve myself at the dinner table, but not seconds. If my Mom forgot to replenish my plate, that was it; I stayed hungry. But I wasn't completely at the mercy of my stupid attitude, because I wasn't completely stupid. I made it my policy to run to the ice box (ice box, not refrigerator) whenever nobody else was around. I have always suspected that my mother's ice box logistics were partly in deference to me and my peculiar personality.

You can understand that I carried this distorted brain and spirit with me wherever I went, including school. "I ain't gonna beg you for nuthin'. If you don't wanna give it to me, the heck with you." And that was how it was for five resentful years. I hated that sick, antisocial, feeling but could do nothing about it. I even knew my mind was sick but I wasn't going to kowtow to these bastards.

I acted the same way with a lovely girl friend whom I truly loved, as teenagers love, anyway. When someone reported to me that she was holding hands with George, that was it. I flat-out dropped her without a word. She wrote me a long impassioned letter, but even though I hurt badly to be near her again, I never answered her. I well knew I wasn't being fair with her but was frozen tight in a mental trap of some kind and couldn't get out of it. That's how sick I was. I only hope she has forgiven me, though she has no good reason to.

In my senior year, lo and behold, I was elected captain of our track team. What in the world...? Well, anyway I was going to be able to participate.

I had long been eager to run the quarter-mile, also known as the 440. A quarter was about my limit, as I had always been plagued by an abnormal lack of endurance. But my long, easy stride made up for my lack. I would just about collapse at the end of a quarter but I knew I could beat anybody in school. Ironically I could not fit my quarter into the schedule, given the other events I was entered in. So I assigned the quarter to someone else and was instead to anchor the mile relay, which featured four runners to run a quarter-mile each. My friend Marcello was to run the lead-off lap in my spiked shoes and then hurriedly take them off during the second and third laps so I could put them on to run the anchor.

My first event was the high jump. While I was still competing in it, a call came over the loudspeaker, "First call for the first heat of the 120-yard low hurdles." In due time, "Third and last call for the first heat of the 120-yard hurdles." Then, "Hey, Bert, get to the starting line or I'll scratch you."

"I'm still jumping. How about moving me over to the second heat?"

"Okay, but you better be ready."

The high jump came down to two remaining jumpers, Chosei and me. We both made it at five-four. Then I missed one at five-five. Then, "Third and final call for the second heat of the 120-yard low hurdles. Bert, if you're not here

19

right now, you're scratched." So I accepted second place in the jump and sprinted over to the starting holes. We didn't have starting blocks or jet-assisted take-offs in those days. We had to scratch our own starting holes in the ground. (Neither did we have sling shots for vaulting poles nor baskets for baseball gloves.) The moment I got there, Bang! We were off and I won my heat by a mile and so qualified for the final heat. "All right fellas, let's get going. We're behind schedule. Get set for the final heat." Another sprint to the starting holes. Bang! Off we went, and you know who ran away from the pack.

Then, "First and last call for the mile relay." I started to take my spikes off for Marcello to run the lead lap. "Excelsiors, we can't wait for you. I'm scratching you from the mile relay."

I had no choice but to tie my spikes back on, take off for the starting holes, and run the lead. Bang! Off we went on the lead lap. Though I was still puffing from all the running I had just done, I was thrilled to be running the quarter mile at last. I was exhilarated as I gradually pulled away from the five others. About a hundred yards from where my partner was waiting to take the baton from me, I switched on my afterburner and started to increase my lead, when Yow! My buttock muscles abruptly cramped. Though I pulled as hard as I could it was impossible to come close to maintaining my pace, and the pain was increasing. Five bodies passed me and I wondered whether I could last long enough to pass the baton. I barely made it and collapsed on the track in great pain. Worse, I had placed my club at least ten yards behind the field. Talk about humiliation! But our speed burners made up part of the deficit and came in second anyway.

Obviously I was disadvantaged by having to run those events in such rapid succession, but I doubt that a "normal" person would have broken down the way I did. But anyway, that was just another sad failure in my life.

Three years after I got out of high school and one year after I flunked out of college, the Catholic Youth Organization sponsored a boxing tournament citywide, with boys of any denomination welcome to compete. Since the rounds in the amateurs were only two minutes long, I wondered whether I should try for it. So I went to Charlie Miller's Gym downtown and started to train, still not sure whether I could build up enough endurance for the ordeal. When you're exhausted in the ring you don't just go home. You either quit in disgrace or you go down in ultimate defeat. You get knocked out. Kayoed. Humiliated! Miller's Gym was a big one, with thirty to forty fighters working out at one time; hitting the bags, sparring in the rings, jumping rope, shadow boxing. One evening while I was working out "pretty good," Danny Gonzales, a prominent fight manager and trainer, walked across the floor and said to me, "Hey, kid, come here." He walked into one of the rings and I followed him. Then he yelled, "Hey, Manny, come here!" Manny was Manuel Bochan, then Hawaii's professional welterweight champion. When Manny got into the ring, Danny told him, "Check this kid out." So Manny checked me out. Holding his hands up with palms toward me, he said, "Throw me a stiff left jab. Throw a straight right. Hard. Hook. Hard." I had only tape on my hands and was sure I was hurting Manny's hands. Then with his orders to hit he started to flick his hands toward my face and sometimes toward my body. So I had to hit, block, bob, hit, sidestep, hit. He picked up the pace and moved side-to-side, in, out, in circles, and to keep up with him I

21

had to step pretty lively. He brought out the best in me and I felt great knowing I was mixing it up with the pro champ. Of course he wasn't hitting me but I felt good anyway. "This kid's got the moves," he said to Danny. "He's a natural."

Danny asked me, "You ever fight before?"

"No."

"You wanna fight pro?"

"If you train me, yeah. Sure, I'll fight pro."

Then to Manny, "We can train him with Chico." Chico was Chico Rosa, whom I had been watching and admiring. He was just seventeen then but beautiful to watch as he bobbed and weaved. What I admired most about him was that he combined his bobbing and weaving with a lot of aggressive hitting, a style employed by the late Jack Dempsey, the great Manassa Mauler. Chico was soon to turn pro and eventually become the world's featherweight champ after defeating the likes of Sandy Saddler, whom old timers may remember as having fought Willie Pep four times as they exchanged the featherweight title between themselves in torrid battles. I looked forward with excitement to training with Chico Rosa.

So there I was, on the threshold of fighting in the fast lane with Danny Gonzales and Manny Bochan to manage and train me. With Chico to boot. I was excited, to say the least. "Follow me." So I followed my future manager. We went to the supply room, where he ordered the attendant, "Give this kid the best shoes you've got." Those shoes were the ultimate, lighter than I ever thought any shoes could be, high-cut and shiny-black. I think they were made of goatskin. When I put them on they felt as though I had nothing on, except that they provided heavenly support for my feet and ankles and helped me to move with greater efficiency.

That same evening I was approached by David Paishon, much better known to oldtimers as Indian, the notorious street fighter. He was supposed to have been a cross between Hawaiian and one of the Hispanic races and tagged with the name Indian because his face was always red from drinking. Anyway, Indian was apparently now well in his forties and considerably mellowed. He asked me, "Hey, Wong, where do you live?"

"Palolo."

"Then you're supposed to fight for me at Saint Patrick's Parish. Why don't you meet me there tomorrow around five? You can help us out a lot."

"Okay, Indian. I'll see you there tomorrow." I didn't think Danny would be needing to see me very soon, so I thought it was okay.

The next evening when I met Indian at Saint Patrick's he gave me the most beautiful pair of boxing trunks I could ever hope to wear. They fit perfectly and were of shiny white satin with a green waistband, green stripes down the sides, and a green shamrock on the front of the left leg. To add glory to the gift, many of the other fighters didn't have the same thing, and with my classy new shoes I felt like a prima donna, almost like a pro already.

Indian ran our training admirably, surprising me with his discipline. I soon found out that not only was he a notorious street fighter but that he also knew a lot about ring fighting, too. He conducted himself and spoke pretty much like a cultured gentleman. I gave him a lot of points.

One of the fellows among us seemed to dislike me, for whatever reason, I don't know. Perhaps he was just the quiet type and perhaps I just read him wrong. Or perhaps

23

he resented my fancy pro outfit. Anyway, I found myself
disliking him in return. One evening Indian said, "Joe, put
on the gloves. Wong, put on the gloves." Joe and I were
going to have a sparring session, but to me we were going
to have it out. Right off, I threw him a straight right to the
face and caught him "real good." He didn't like that and
was obviously bent on getting back even. I caught him
with another straight right, this time to the gut. I feinted
another right to his gut and then switched to a wicked
overhand right to his face. If you have ever fought much,
you may know how much of your bodyweight you can add
to an overhand blow, especially with enough elbow behind
it. That's what I did, and Whop! It landed on Joe's left
eyebrow and opened up a horrible cut, dropping blood to
the floor in a few seconds. I was surprised that the twelve-
ounce pillows we were using were capable of such damage,
but then maybe Manny was right when he said I had the
moves. Joe was furious and started to charge in retaliation.
But he was such a pathetic sight that I just couldn't continue
hitting him, and so just kept backing away until Indian
called a halt to the melee. Poor Joe. I felt very sorry and
found myself liking him, but I never saw him again.

At St. Patrick's we trained in the school auditorium, a
sterile environment not quite appropriate for fight training.
So the following week I went to train at the Miller gym
again, just for a change of pace, to see some of the friends I
had made there, and just because I missed the historical
old gym with its ingrained fragrances of sweat and liniment.
Anyway, who should approach me, very obviously furious,
but my manager-to-be. Danny half-yelled at me. "Where
the hell you been all week! I've been looking all over hell
for you!"

"Indian told me I had to fight for St. Patrick."

"I thought you were going to fight for Cathedral."

"Myself, I don't care which club I fight for. Anyway, I didn't think I was going to work out with you 'til after the tournament."

Danny looked at me for quite a while, then said, "If you don't wanna work out with me, gimme back my (expletive) shoes!" Off came my beloved shoes and back to my former manager-to-be.

I was so disappointed that I never again aspired to fighting, and never again worked out in a fight gym. Why did I give up with Danny so easily? I probably could have talked my way back into his good graces, and I really think he half-expected and half-wanted me to try. But since I didn't demonstrate the guts to defend myself, he probably gave up on me too. But I chickened out for a couple of good reasons: First, as so often happened in the past, my thinking process went blank and I didn't know what to say and how to say it. Second, the well-founded fear of not being able to get into shape had haunted me and prevented me from developing any kind of resolve in this endeavor. I couldn't get properly warmed up. Instead of sweating, I got nauseated and chilled. Of course the doctors didn't know a gnat's pimple about such things. I got pretty dubious whenever I thought about fighting four three-minute rounds as a pro, let alone ten torrid rounds if I ever got that far. But this was nothing new for me. It was absurd anyway to have even entertained the prospect of even stepping into a fight ring. My bad health had always roadblocked me seemingly in everything I undertook. But life goes on, perhaps not exactly how we would like it to, but it goes on. All the same, I wondered what unknown cause it was that kept me in generally poor condition, both physically and mentally. Perhaps some day I would find out. Perhaps.

I once played and enjoyed golf, but only for three years until our first child was born and I switched to washing diapers, making formula, walking the floor, and such. Most of it was just informal play on the way home from work, but I did play in a couple tournaments. Though not winning a prize of any kind, some of my play was spectacular and well worth discussing here, because my same old malady did me in again. My first tournament was an inter-shop affair at the Pearl Harbor Naval Shipyard, one 18-hole round played on each of four consecutive Saturdays at different courses. The first Saturday I one-putted the first hole. The second Saturday I one-putted the first hole. The third Saturday my approach shot landed six inches short of the green. My partner Roy "Corky" Porter tried to console me. "Sorry, Bert, you ain't gonna one-putt this one."

I said, "Well, let's see."

"Impossible. It's a 50-footer, and to play that slope you'll have to go off the green and then you'll roll down that steep apron."

"Roy, I told you, 'Let's see.'"

"You'll see. I see already. You're good but you can't do the impossible."

"The impossible will take a little longer." I was parroting the slogan of the Shipyard during the war. The ball rolled to the very edge of the green before turning in and rolling into the cup. I had one-putted the first hole again, the third time in three consecutive rounds. Roy fell to the ground, not to mention the reactions of our two opponents.

The next round was played on the Mid-Pacific Country Club course in Lanikai. Our foursome started play on the tenth hole. On this one most golfers had to baby their drive, because a long one would land in a deep gully in front of the green. For some stupid reason I topped my second shot and landed in the bottom of that gully. The three others pitched over the gully onto the green. From the gully I pitched my third shot into the hole. Despite a flubbed shot I still got a birdie on that hole and didn't have to putt at all, depriving myself of the opportunity to run my string of first-hole one-putters to four.

The only other tournament round I played was between the Fort Shafter Golf Club, my home club, and an outfit from Schofield Barracks, another Army post. I one-putted the first four holes and was three under par at that point. I did the front nine in 34, one under par, and the back nine in 48. This was the first and last time I ever played the back nine under 50 on any course.

Now, what has all this got to do with health? An awful lot. Rather it was my state of health that had a lot to do with my golf. I always started out like a pro and ended up like a duffer. My energy and concentration were always okay at the start but always faded as play progressed. The front nine was usually done in the low 40's, occasionally in the high 30's, and the back nine in the 50's. I recall always trying to bear down in the latter part of the round but running out of energy in body and mind. I just could not handle the job.

To summarize: In the five tournament rounds of golf I ever played, I one-putted the first hole four times, one-putted the first four holes in succession once, and pitched into the first hole once without having to putt. That looks like sensational professional golf to anybody, but my total scores were mediocre at best. This was because my play consistently deteriorated as I continued to play and run out of energy.

Let's look at a couple more examples of how lack of physical and mental energy can affect one's endeavors.

In 1979 I got into the silver market and ran my account to $2,000,000. With a margin loan of $470,000, my equity was a bit over $1-1/2 million. As usually happens, I lost my concentration, let my surveillance slip, and lost the entire account and then some, ending up with a debt to my broker. Same old story.

More recently, I decided to make a pile of money in the commodity futures market and opened an account with $6000. Being very much in earnest, I set up a special office for the project, installing a new telephone in the room, making pigeonholes for the paperwork, and subscribed to chart services. So intent was I in my work that I spent about six hours a day in that office, much of it on the telephone. In exactly ninety days I had a profit of $47,000. That's a 783 percent profit, or 3133 percent per annum. But the same old bugaboo snuck in again and I found it increasingly difficult to concentrate on my project. I just couldn't stand analyzing those complicated charts anymore. I had lost the power to concentrate. In a few weeks I lost almost all my profits. Same old story. Ho hum...

This deterioration of concentration and performance is the story of my life. Shortage of health, shortage of energy. Shortage of energy, shortage of results. Auspicious beginning, ignominious end. At those times, without a legitimate and extenuating excuse to console me, I simply felt like a no-good failure.

In early 1941, mobilizing for possible war, the U.S. Navy conducted a test for candidates seeking apprenticeship positions at their shipyard, then officially called the Pearl Harbor Navy Yard. About 800 boys from all over Hawaii took the test and I came in first with a score of 98.08. So I had my choice of trades and decided to go into pattern-making. No, not dressmaking. Patternmaking is a little-known but highly respected trade. A patternmaker makes forms for the molder, who uses these forms, called patterns, to make sand molds into which is poured molten metal to make castings of items such as pumps, valves, brackets of all kinds, engine blocks, cylinder heads, impellers, propellers, and anything else that had to be in the form of a casting. At that time the "benchmark" journeymen like the machinist, electrician, shipfitter, and sheetmetal worker at Pearl were getting $1.17 an hour; the patternmaker was getting $1.41. But his job is stressful. Thinking in the abstract is a very integral part of his duties.

I became an apprentice patternmaker, with my supervisors expecting great performance from me, the number one qualifier. Well, to tell you honestly, I was not a standout at all. I guess I did all right but had a serious flaw. My sick mind still had me in its grip. I did fine work and my products were decorator pieces, accurately dimensioned and beautifully varnished. But my speed suffered terribly, and in time of war speed was infinitely more valuable than flawless accuracy and immaculate appearance. This was such a problem that my supervisor often spoke to me about it. "Bert, it doesn't have to be that pretty. The ship is waiting for the part." I always agreed and promised to try my best to be more practical. However, my "obsessive-compulsive" nature would not allow me to put out anything but the highest-quality work. I knew I was not the asset to the Navy that I wanted to be. Whether my sick body was making my mind sick or was it the other way around I didn't know. But no matter; I was sick. Ever see a person who was nervous and sleepy at the same time? That was what I was. I often wished I could sink into the floor and disappear. Not only that; I got into three fights in my Civil Service career. Of course I was always in the right (Ask me; I'll tell you.), but how does one justify three fights when millions of employees work long years without a single fight? Was there something wrong with me? Ha!

Three months before our marriage in 1944 everything seemed to go wrong with my body and mind. I was extremely nervous, ravenously hungry, losing weight, confused, weak, gassy, and had a never-ending headache. Often I was awake all night with a fast pulse. After our marriage I tried to fix up the home we had bought but made very slow progress, being stymied by the simplest tasks. My mind and body were in turmoil, and I was at a complete loss as to how to pull them out. I had three big-time boils. I was getting weaker and could feel my insides quiver.

I don't recall how many doctors I visited or how many tests I underwent, but they were many, and every one was useless. Of course the words "hypochondria" and "psychosomatic" inevitably came up. One doctor hesitatingly asked if I were willing to go see a psychiatrist. I said, "If you think I should go, of course I'll go." He told me whom to go to and I went straight to his office to make an appointment. I spoke to his receptionist just long enough to make an appointment and then left. In a couple days I received a bill for $15, for making an appointment at the front desk. That was in 1945, and that $15 was probably like $150 today. I surmised that part of the take went back to the doctor who referred me. Even then those M.D.s had things pretty well set up. I paid the thirty pieces of silver and canceled the appointment.

In almost complete hopelessness I tried to accept my unhappy state and live with it. But I was miserable and more confused than ever. There was no way I could live indefinitely with the headaches, gas, hunger, nervousness, insomnia, boils, hay fever, ad infinitum. Everybody pitied

30

me. The only way I could walk without staggering too much was to walk extra fast. Every day my lunch can weighed a ton, loaded down with nothing but heavy carbohydrates: peanut butter and jelly sandwiches, cake, puddings, candy, and such. I left out the vacuum bottle, because it took up valuable space that could be used for more valued sweet stuff. I ate throughout the day and of course my supervisors frowned on that.

One day a friend said to me, "There's a doctor on Nuuanu Avenue who might be able to help you. He's an old man from Japan and he's not very fluent in English. Maybe you'd like to go see him."

"In my condition I have no choice. I'll go see anybody. Where is his place and what is his name?"

My friend gave me the particulars and I went to see the old man, who was a regularly licensed physician. He said, "Good morning. What is wrong?"

"I don't know what is wrong, because a hundred doctors don't know. So I cannot answer you."

"All right. What is symptom?"

"Not symptom. Many symptoms: hunger, nervousness, headaches, insomnia, mental confusion..."

Dr. Mori interrupted. "I think is no trouble. Perhaps you have hypoglycemia."

"What is hypoglycemia?"

"It is related to diabetes. If you take care now, not serious. But if you neglect, it will become diabetes. But do not worry. I think we can take care. Give me specimen, please." He handed me a glass beaker. When I returned it to him with the specimen he added a few drops of something in it, then warmed it over a Bunsen burner. "Yes, you have hypoglycemia. But do not worry, I will help you. If you follow instructions you will be all right." Then he went to his desk drawer and produced a Ditto sheet of instructions specifically for hypoglycemia. "You follow instructions carefully, please. If you still have trouble come back again. But I think you will not have to come back."

I thought, "If Dr. Mori has these sheets all made up specifically for hypoglycemia and ready to give to his patients, this can't be such a rare disease." So I asked him. "Is this a rare disease?"

"No. Many people have."

"Then why haven't my other doctors told me about it? Do they know what it is?"

"They don't like to say," He seemed to be at a loss for the right words.

"They don't like to say what? That they don't know? That they know?"

"They say, 'No such thing. Superstition.'"

"What do you think about it?"

"Nothing to think. In other country many people have hypoglycemia. In United States nobody have hypoglycemia. But many people have hypoglycemia." Dr. Mori seemed to be bent on being discreet in saying what he wanted to say.

"You seem to be saying that American doctors don't want to diagnose hypoglycemia. Why is that?"

Dr. Mori seemed reluctant to discuss the matter but I sensed that, being such a nice person, neither did he want to rebuff a patient sincerely in search of vital information. So he answered, "Very inexpensive to treat hypoglycemia. Not very easy for patient but not expensive. If treatment successful, no more doctor bill. No more money."

"Dr. Mori, are you telling me that American doctors prefer to keep their patients sick so they will keep coming back for more testing and consultations they would not need if they were correctly diagnosed?"

"No. I don't tell anything. Not my business. You go home think for yourself. Please you give me ten dollars. Go home follow instruction sheet. You will be all right."

I left Dr. Mori's office disturbedly ambivalent. I felt enlightened and yet could not quite believe that my doctors would let me suffer so terribly for two long years just so they could make a few more dollars. How could anyone, especially a doctor, be so cruel? What about all the other years of my life? Could hypoglycemia been responsible for all that misery too? Maybe they truly didn't know about the disease. But how could they not know about such an apparently simple disease? Maybe they didn't, and don't want to know. A-a-a-ah!

At home I studied Dr. Mori's instructions and shortly began to put them to use. In a surprisingly short time I began to feel a distinct difference in my physical condition. I also sensed that my mind was more tranquil. I was convinced of my improvement when I happily noticed that I wasn't clenching my teeth as hard and as often as before, and with that my tension headaches were mitigating. My hunger was getting less desperate and demanding. I was getting much more needed sleep. It wasn't long before there was no more doubt. I was getting well and was exhilarated! In a few months I was close to being in normal health. But Dr. Mori had told me that a hypoglycemic would always be a hypoglycemic and that I would have to be on my toes for life as far as my diet was concerned.

You know of course that I did a lot of high-powered thinking for a while. I also often shook my head in disbelief. How could conditions be the way they seemed to be? If the doctors actually did not know about hypoglycemia, then somebody's guilty of willful negligence. Questions, questions, questions. I may not have gotten all the answers

33

but I have learned pretty much which end is up and which end is up-side-down. Not only which end; also who is up-side-down and getting it in the end.

As I continued to improve I was almost incredulous that one little simple visit to a comparatively obscure semi-retired doctor of foreign origin could make me feel better than I had felt in my entire life. It was also almost impossible to believe that hypoglycemia was well known in foreign countries but virtually unknown by American doctors, products of the great medical schools in which ambitious foreign medical students aspire to enroll. Even notwithstanding what Dr. Mori alluded to about American doctors, I did not want to believe what appeared to be a certainty. So I put the question on a back burner and turned it down to simmer. More insight would probably develop after a bit more cooking.

In 1946 I enlisted in the Army with two friends. All three of us got perfect scores in the standard 50-question Army enlistment examination. The Captain Lee who administered the test told me three years later that no other enlistee had ever got a perfect score on the test in the many years he administered it. He facetiously wondered whether we had cheated.

I got a score of 143 in the Army General Classification Test (AGCT), which was an intelligence/aptitude test. As in IQ tests, average was 100. Basic training at Camp Lee, Virginia, was tough but tolerable. My health was as good as it had ever been, though that's not saying much.

Toward the end of Basic I was ordered to take the examination for Officer's Candidate School (OCS), which I did. My score was 140 and I was highly recommended for OCS. I accepted the appointment as an Officer Candidate and was sent to Fort Bragg, N.C., with eleven other

Candidates to await assignment to the various training schools. Eventually the eleven were all called and sent to their respective schools. I still had not been called, because the school of my choice was full and not calling for new trainees at that time. It was in Air Force Administration, headquartered at Fort Riley, Kansas, and a field I considered a good place to be in future civilian life. I stuck with my choice because I knew I would not enjoy being in the Infantry or the Artillery, or any of the other choices I had either. The colonel overseeing the program strongly urged me to respond to a call from the Medical School, but I declined that one too, as I had lost my taste for things medical, notwithstanding that at one time in my naive youth I had aspired to being a medicine man. My inability to study was probably what kept me from being a doctor. Again we see that there's often a silver lining to whatever befalls us.

One day the colonel called me in and expressed displeasure over my "obstinacy" in holding out for the school which was oversubscribed and not needing any more trainees. Since I was the only Candidate left under his wing, I felt he was eager to get the program over with. Taking advantage of this assumption I forthwith dropped out of the program, giving him an ostensible reason. But the true reason was the same one which had plagued me all my life: lack of energy and endurance. While waiting for the call from Fort Riley I had been doing a lot of running in an attempt to get into shape. But I could not overcome the inability to sweat. All I did when I pushed myself was get nauseated, chills, and headaches. Singlemindedness was not the prevailing condition. Too, my friend Al Fisher, one of the eleven who were now in the "Ninety-Day-Wonder" training at OCS, was writing me occasionally to let me

35

know how he was faring and to give me perspective on what to expect when I got there. "The rigors of the training are excruciating and quite a few of the fellas are dropping out. Bert, I strongly advise you to get into tip-top shape before starting OCS." That was enough to help me decide. At least I knew I had tried. But the thought occurred to me that this was not my first drop-out.

Though my health wasn't doing very well, inasmuch as hypoglycemia supposedly never leaves one completely unmolested, I did fabulously well as a cook, also known in the Army as a slum burner. The first day of Food Service School, as part of the curriculum I was assigned full charge of the evening meal for the 300 Student Cooks and Bakers in our company. The next morning I was pulled out of the training program and immediately assigned to active duty as First Cook. My rise in rank was nothing short of phenomenal, and as a 15-month veteran of the Army I was the equivalent of a Staff Sergeant. At 24 months I was appointed Operations Sergeant of a new Food Service School, being responsible for the curricula of about 300 Student Cooks and Bakers and the duties of 31 Instructors. Concurrently I was put in for a promotion to Master Sergeant. Ironically, unfortunately, and disappointingly, just around that time, July of 1948, the New Army Career Plan was instituted and promotions were geared to a time table, which made me ineligible not only for the two-step promotion but also for a one-step promotion to Sergeant First Class, formerly known as Technical Sergeant. Since all the other members of the staff were comparative old timers in the Army, having been selected from the ranks of Mess Sergeants to staff the new school, almost every one of them was already, or soon became, a Master Sergeant with the creation of the school. We looked like a herd of zebras whenever we got together. So there I was, a "principal" of a large school and outranked by all the instructors under my supervision. That was enough for me to decide that my first enlistment would be my last.

There was one consolation, however. I was in fair health and my mind seemed somewhat stable. At least I was operating normally enough.

A few months later my mother became critically ill in Hawaii and the Red Cross arranged to have me transferred home. There being no Food Service School in Hawaii at that time, I returned to cooking at Fort Shafter, headquarters of USARPAC, United States Army Pacific. My second day on the job a sergeant came into my kitchen and asked me, "Are you Sergeant Wong?"

"Yes, I am."

"General Aurand would like you to be his personal cook," Lieutenant General Henry Aurand wore three stars and was Chief of Staff of USARPAC, the entire Pacific area.

"Does General Aurand want me or does Personnel want to assign me?"

"I said General Aurand wants you."

"How in hell does he know anything about me? I just got here yesterday fresh from South Carolina."

"His staff members know about you. Some of them came from Fort Jackson too."

"I guess that makes me a world-famous Army slumburner."

"Yes, you're famous all right. Do you want to cook for the general or not? You and your wife will live in the large house directly behind his mansion on Palm Circle. You will be promoted to Sergeant First Class and receive an extra hundred dollars a month in your pay. But you will have to re-enlist, since you're slated for discharge next

37

month. I suggest you accept this offer, Sergeant Wong. General Aurand is a wonderful man, a kind you won't meet every day. Think about it and I'll ask you again tomorrow."

Though my old job in Pearl Harbor's highest-paying shop was awaiting my return, I was tempted to take the General up on his offer, not so much for the promotion and extra pay, but because General Aurand was roundly known and respected for his high level of intelligence and capabilities. I knew we would become good friends. Also, because my wife was employed by the Army as a secretary and had good credentials, I was sure the General would be a definite asset to her career. Nevertheless, after due consideration I reluctantly decided to decline the offer and return to Pearl to resume my job as a patternmaker. I told the Personnel sergeant my decision.

A few days later I went on sick call for a back problem and was told summarily that it was all in my head. So I got a bright idea and went straight to the Neuropsychiatric Clinic of the Tripler General Hospital and got myself admitted to Ward 27, where psychosomatic cases were studied and treated. Great! I had always been intrigued by the mind. But in two weeks I was told that my back injury was confirmed but that it should improve with time. I was to be discharged soon. I was disappointed, because I was having the proverbial ball, a well deserved vacation after three years of hard and faithful service to Uncle Sam. I asked my ward doctor if he could somehow get the decision reversed and keep me there a bit longer. He said he would try and the next day surprised me by saying I could stay. I wondered how in the world this lieutenant could pull it off, until I was told later that a Captain Toombs had a hand in the reversal. Captain Toombs was coach of the Tripler softball team in the USARPAC league and apparently had been watching us play in the inter-ward games. He asked me and Bill Fitzgerald, another patient, to play for the cadre team, me at second base and Bill at third. I think Bill and I justified the captain's faith in us. In one game the batter of the opposing team hit a pop-fly foul 'way off the first-base line. The first baseman and the catcher made a try for it but gave up, because it was too far out of reach. Plop! Bill Fitzgerald the third baseman got it!

In another game I got two hits while nobody else on our team got any, thus saving us from being the victims of a no-hitter. In fast-pitch softball hits are not easy to come by, as fast-pitch players well know. In the next game I got another while Bill got one and nobody else got any. I was batting around .470.

I stole third a couple times, and on one of the steals the opposing coach bawled the catcher out so vehemently that the catcher threw down his mask and went home. In softball the runner is not allowed to leave a base until the catcher has the ball in his mitt. So base stealing is not so much a matter of speed but more of strategy and deception. What allowed me to be so aggressive, I felt, was the superior physical, mental, and spiritual health I was enjoying as a result of healthful living. The cafeteria-style food service was just what the doctor had ordered (Dr. Mori, that is, in 1945, four years before.) and I found great joy in observing the discipline of a good hypoglycemic diet. Being free of duty responsibilities helped too. I got to go to the beach every day on the hospital bus if I wanted to. With the softball activities I was getting enough exercise. Then every Tuesday night I jumped on the hospital bus and went to see the professional fights free at the Civic Auditorium or the Honolulu Stadium. In Occupational Therapy we could make just about anything we wanted to, and all materials were free; free to us anyway if not to the taxpayer. Thank you.

In further enhancement of my racket I was allowed to spend every weekend at home with my wife. This was the life of Riley, a super vacation. The seven months I spent at Tripler were some of the happiest in my life, made more enjoyable by the comparison to the difficulties of my life in general. In December of 1949 I was discharged from Tripler, but my experience there had a lot to do with how I feel about health today.

In 1952 we had our first child, a boy. By that time I had allowed the cares of daily living to distract me from the discipline of prudent living. All three of us were not very healthy. I did not recognize that my hypoglycemia had come back on me, because the symptoms were not nearly like the ones that had hit me before. But sick was sick, and that was what I was. Sinusitis pained me so much that I visited an Eye, Ear, Nose and Throat specialist every now and then for a medicinal irrigation. Those were bloody events. On one of the visits Dr. Maurice Gordon said to me, "Why are you not coming for treatments as often as I ask you to?"

"Well," I said, "for one thing that needle of yours hurts so much and aggravates the inside of my nose so much that it nullifies the benefits of the irrigation. Two, how long is this treatment going to take, anyway?"

"How long is what going to take?"

"Well, what am I coming here for?"

"Are you thinking of curing your sinusitis?"

"Isn't that what we're trying to do?"

"No, no, no. Nobody ever cured sinusitis."

"Then what are we trying to do?"

"Minimizing your misery and trying to keep you happier."

With that I stopped going to Dr. Gordon and went to

another specialist. I asked him, "Do you plan to cure my sinusitis?"

Dr. Andrew Wong smiled and said, "Well, I've never cured anybody else's sinusitis and frankly I don't think I can cure yours."

Woe was me, as they say. Was I going to have to live with this misery all my life? Fortuitously, just about that time I received in the mail a free sample of Prevention Magazine, which was a somewhat new health publication. They said, "Send us eighty cents and we'll send you the next ten issues." So I subscribed.

I liked so much what I read that I was inspired to take drastic action. I went to our kitchen and, over my wife's protestations, tossed out much of what had passed as food: cola drinks, cookies, candy, potato chips, sugar, ice cream, ad nauseum. I borrowed my mother's Sweden Speed Juicer and we drank fresh juices, both fruit and vegetable. We ate mostly fresh, live food. No artificial, unnatural sugar of any kind, white, brown, or raw. No white bread or any other pastries. As I said, the action was drastic, so inspired was I and so desperate to extricate myself from the terrible feeling of illness.

As I had been admonished by Prevention's introductory literature not to expect immediate results in health, I was very pleasantly surprised, indeed exhilarated, when we all began to feel better in a few days, not cured by any means but recognizably better. I had been the sickest of us three, and so my improvement was the most dramatic. My nose stopped running, my sinuses cleared up and stopped hurting, my cold hands and feet warmed up, my joints hurt much less, and I just felt much better all around. Our little boy stopped coughing. My wife's cold cleared up. I don't recall how fast we improved but it was surprisingly fast. That was 1954.

People being what they are, we tend to take things for granted when things go right, and that is what I did. In 1964 and 1965 I was very sick again. I weighed 117 pounds in my street clothes. I don't know why I didn't suspect the return of hypoglycemia; I just didn't. After several visits to my internist he said, "Look, Bert, I can't do anything for you. You'll have to do it for yourself, because you're making yourself sick. You know why you're so skinny and nervous? Because your mind is nervous, and your mind is nervous because you've got the cares of the world on your shoulders. Go home and quit worrying over everything and you'll be all right."

I said, "You're saying my troubles are psychosomatic. I say they're somatopsychotic. I may not be a doctor but I know my body is making my mind sick, not the other way around."

"Oh, go home and forget about it. I told you I can't help you."

"Are you saying you give up on me?"

He gave me a very condescending smile and pushed me toward the door. "Just quit chasing shadows and you'll get well."

Well, I was on my own again. One day I read about a book entitled "Body, Mind and Sugar" and it piqued my interest. I ordered it in hopes it would give me some insight into health and sickness. And that it did. It was all about hypoglycemia and it was about me. What, again? Responding to the authors' recommendation, I went to the Occidental Laboratory and requested a six-hour glucose tolerance test. "Okay," the receptionist said. "Where's the prescription?"

"What prescription?"

"For your test. Don't you have one? We can't give you a test without a prescription. It's the law."

I thought, "These guys really have this racket all sewed up. Aren't they getting enough money from us yet? Another visit to the doctor and another bill." But I said, "Okay. I'll go get one."

Back I went to my former internist. As soon as I walked into his office he said, "What? You still worrying about your health?"

"No. I'm going to fix myself up."

"Then what are you doing here?"

"I just want one thing from you: a prescription for a six-hour glucose tolerance test."

"Oh, for crying out loud! You probably think you have hypoglycemia. Don't waste your time listening to that stuff. It's just a fad."

"If you won't give me the prescription I'll go next door and get it from Dr. Richard."

"Okay, okay. Sit down. He wrote and handed me a prescription. It prescribed a three-hour test.

"Hey, I need a six-hour test."

"Who the hell is the doctor, anyway? The three-hour test is standard."

"I know, and that's why your poor patients aren't being diagnosed right. I'll go next door."

"Dammit, Bert. Sit down! If you want a six-hour test I'll prescribe one, but I don't know what for. Here. Bring the results to me, okay?"

"What the heck for? You gave up on me, remember? So I'm fixing myself up, and I don't need you."

"Come on, Bert. Don't be so stubborn. Bring the report back, okay?"

"Okay, but I don't know what for."

When I took the test I almost lost consciousness in the last hour, a typical reaction of the advanced hypoglycemic that I was. Now finally, thanks to the thorough explanation in "Body, Mind and Sugar," I felt confident that I knew the cause of my decades of misery. In fact I was already on the recommended corrective diet, which was similar to the one recommended to me by Dr. Mori twenty years before. Nevertheless, I took the test report to my internist as promised.

He looked at the report, then looked at it again. "You've got a bad case of hypoglycemia."

"Yeah, yeah, I told you about it. Now we both know. Okay. Thanks. Be seeing you."

"Wait a second. I'm not through with you yet. I'm putting you on a diet."

"No, you're not. I'm already on a diet."

"You know what to do?"

"Of course. You told me I had to do it for myself, so I did it."

"Okay, okay. Tell me what you're doing."

I told him the details of my diet and he seemed to agree. He said, "Stick with your diet and come back six months from now. I want to test you again."

I managed a sigh of impatience with this doctor who had insisted there was nothing wrong with me except my head. Perhaps I was rubbing it in too much. So I said, "Okay. See you in six months."

Six months later we went through the same routine, this time without argument. The test showed me to be in good shape. Not only that; I had gained a few pounds. After studying the report the doctor said, "You son-of-a-bitch! You diagnosed and cured your own case."

"Thanks a lot."

As Dr. Robert C. Atkins says, "A knowledgeable patient can make his doctor a wise man."

I presume you understand why I don't mention the names of certain characters in these stories.

Not much later, during the Vietnam war, I accepted a position at the U.S. Naval Ship Repair Facility on Guam. While there I made about a dozen trips to Vietnam, Thailand, and the Philippines to inspect their naval vessels as well as some of our own. The average length of each visit was about ten days. On two of the trips I went alone. On the others about a dozen of us went. Six of the trips were to Vietnam.

Now here's something that has a lot to do with one of the major theses of this book. On these trips it was the standing rule that we were to drink only special bottled water and never to eat except at the military establishments or at our hotel, and this was because we knew that ol' Confucius was always ready to take out his revenge on us. Still, seemingly without fail some members of our group always complained about their reaction to the food and water. But I was never troubled by the problem, and this was not because I was lucky. There was a very specific reason for it. The diet I had adopted to keep my hypoglycemia at bay was in fact a pretty good diet for general health for anybody. It promoted freedom from debris in the blood and tissues. When one's body is clean in and out, bugs don't bother him and he doesn't get infections. I'll explain this concept in detail a bit later when we discuss metabolic cleanliness. For now I'll relate an episode to further illustrate how well the idea works.

45

(We're back on Guam now.) One morning when I came in to work before seven, my boss Dick Dyer said, "Hey, Bert, don't even sit down. Get all the plans and data for the Vietnamese Command Center job, go home, pack your luggage, and take off for Andersen (Air Force Base). Your flight is scheduled. You have a 5 p.m. appointment with Commander (So-and-So) at Fleet Command in Saigon." So I flew to Saigon and met with the American Commander at five. We discussed and planned the project until 9:30 p.m. and I was weak and nervous with hunger, as I hadn't had a thing to eat since lunch on the plane. (Remember, "Once a hypoglycemic, always a hypoglycemic.") The Navy driver dropped me at my hotel and I eagerly looked forward to my ten o'clock dinner. Well, the dining room had already closed down for the evening. Those military hotels didn't cater to late-night dinners. So I went down to the street with intentions of finding an Officers' Mess open. No luck. The streets were absolutely dead. I had forgotten about the curfew. Fortunately, on my way out I had noticed one of those push-carts that peddled noodles. But we never ate at those places, because sanitation was absolutely nil there. They had no running water and dish washing consisted of dipping the customer's used bowl into an old galvanized pail of a gray liquid that had once been water. The idea seemed to be that the next serving of boiling-hot soup would kill the remaining germs. It seemed that the system worked for the Vietnamese anyway. Whatever the case, I had no choice at all in the matter. I'd either eat noodles right then and there or go crazy or faint from hunger and nervousness. So I ordered. The old man had had a long day and was tapering off his operations. The soup was slightly warm, not even hot enough to be appetizing and obviously not hot enough to kill any germs. As I finished off a second bowlful and headed back to the hotel I thought, "Let's see what ol' Confucius can do with me. Nothing, I bet. I'm too tough for him." Sure enough, nothing happened. I flew back to Guam as healthy as I was when I had left.

I should tell you that I didn't learn a thing from that episode about resistance to germs. I had learned that long before. Here is how this thing works: It is not only what you have just consumed that determines whether you suffer some gastrointestinal infection. It is also what you have eaten in the past and how you have cared for your health and durability — your internal cleanliness and strength. Contaminated food taken into a clean, well-nourished body sometimes is not enough to support the proliferation of microbes. Sometimes it's not the foreign water; it's your way of life.

In fact, I haven't had any kind of flu since 1954. Before that I seemed to catch everything that "went around," as well as some that didn't. Now I never catch colds under normal, typical, conditions. In these 43 years I've caught four colds, every one under unusual and extenuating conditions. For example: I once went on a whole-grain kick, eating bowls of whole-grain wheat and millet. We health nuts do get a bit exuberant at times. My stomach couldn't take all that roughage so abruptly and developed a fever and then a heavy cold.

Three years ago I secluded myself in Guadalajara, Mexico, to write this book. (See how much I love you?) Before I left Tennessee several friends said, "Don't eat the local food. Be sure to take a big bottle of Pepto Bismol with you."

In Guadalajara a Norte Americano doctor originally from New York who had lived in Mexico nineteen years addressed a group of us Gringos, members of the American Society,

47

and one of his pieces of advice was, "Never eat any raw vegetables in Mexico. Cook all vegetables!"

I thought to myself (I never think to anyone else.), "Here we go again. How sad that so many people must live in such fear of the wonderful food given to us so generously by a loving Creator." To me this borders on superstition. All right, then let's call it semi-superstition. The way modern Americans live, yes indeed, they had better be afraid of germs. But the silly superstition is that they think it is normal for germs to attack healthy bodies. We'll talk more about our little friends a bit later.

In my eight weeks in Mexico I ate lots and lots of raw salads. I ate some great tacos at the littlest, folksiest, lunch stands. I also bought a kilo of shelled pumpkin seeds right out of an open bin. My Mexican landlady chided me for my carelessness, saying that even some local folks shy away from such places. Was I a foolish boy, a brave soul? Not at all. You see, I knew that Montezuma knew that he'd just be wasting his time even looking at me. To be more succinct about this, no, I have never gotten sick from eating the local food in foreign lands. And I've been on every continent except Australia. Neither would you have to fear the little dears if you would keep your body reasonably free of junk.

It used to be that whenever I cut myself or otherwise opened up my flesh, I festered and got infections just like "normal" people. But since 1954, I have never applied anything to my wounds, and I heal much faster than I used to. I have tried to maintain a kinship with all life.

It is noteworthy that even when I had those intermittent spells of bad health due to hypoglycemia, I never got infections. The explanation to that is that all the refined sugar, including brown, that I have consumed since 1954 could probably be stuffed into a small teacup. That alone will keep your blood and tissues much cleaner than "normal."

Let me relate to you yet another experience which should not only interest but also perhaps benefit you. This concerns Mexico, so I'll take a short respite from things practical and approach the subject by way of a very passing description of our neighbor country. Contrary to the popular concept in the United States, Mejico (I enjoy using that authentic spelling.) is not just one big desert covered with cactus. In fact I was never able to find Pepito sitting or lying in the shade of a cactus under a sombrero and serape, with his little burro nearby. But I did see two donkeys while there, and almost all the serapes I saw were of polyester and hanging in tourist-oriented shops. The country is covered with majestic mountain peaks and canyons. Guadalajara, Mejico's second-largest city where I lived the two months, has a population of about five million, about the same as that of the state of Tennessee. Despite the mile-high altitude of Guadalajara, allergy hit me hard almost as soon as I arrived there. I contemplated returning home to Tennessee where I would be better able to counteract the misery. Before I managed to come to a decision on this, however, I came upon something entitled "The One-Day Miracle Allergy Cure." Oh my goodness. There they go again with their exaggerations and miracles. But without any other promising solutions I decide to try the advice of the author, except that I wasn't going to be so naive as to expect to turn my allergy around in one day. So I went on a three-day green vegetable juice fast. I think it was the second or third day that I began to feel a definite improvement in how I felt. I kept improving and in a few more days all symptoms were gone and never came back. I hasten to add that while the juice fast was essential to my relief, I did something unusual to enhance the speed of the results. And that was a very effective breathing exercise. Now, I had never assigned much value to breathing exercises, thinking them wimpish measures at best and not effective enough to warrant my time and effort. I preferred activities such as pumping iron and slugging it out toe-to-toe with someone. But I had tried the breathing stuff at home before going to Mejico and found it to be of recognizable value, and so decided to give it a chance to see if it could at least alleviate my allergy symptoms. And did it ever! Now I intend to keep breathing exercises an important part of my health regime. I also hasten to add that I dislike telling such stories, because I am just as fed up as you are with exaggerated tales of miraculous recoveries. But I must tell you that the symptoms of my allergy did abate and that I remained in Guadalajara for the planned two months.

I am eager to tell you more about breathing when we discuss it further in the treatise on exercise.

I have told you a whole string of unhappy stories, unhappy for me anyway. But they don't have to be a big waste, because I have learned much from them. And to the extent that I succeed in my endeavor to share the knowledge, my woes will have been worthwhile. So let us glean what we can from my experiences. For one thing, I have given you a sample of how you can be deceived by the medical industry, either by design or through ignorance, both theirs and yours. Should you feel that in this respect I am excessively critical of the medicine men, it appears that you have lived an idyllic life on a remote tropical island.

I have discussed hypoglycemia only because that is what affected, and still affects, me. But don't think this is of no concern of yours. In a practical sense, it is representative of

50

many of the other symptoms many of us suffer, because it is just one of the numerous symptoms of that one disease that is the only disease that befalls us. Further, it is a required condition for many other symptoms. For example, take chronic fatigue syndrome. Until I see evidence to the contrary, I will continue to believe that it is synonymous with hypoglycemia. If they're not the same thing, they at least share many characteristics. I do not believe that chronic fatigue syndrome can exist without hypoglycemia. So for now let's forget about hypoglycemia and call it simply disease.

Another concept I want to impress on you is the body-mind connection. You are an intimate integration of all your parts, including your mind and emotions. Do not entertain the idea that your mind is just an ethereal "something" without a physical basis or cause. Without a body you just don't have a mind. A healthy body nurtures a healthy mind.

Did you notice as I spun all those sorry tales of my non-accomplishments that I always petered out after an auspicious start? In my grade school days that was called by several different names; like lack of ambition, lack of perseverance, lack of stick-to-itiveness, lack of follow-through, laziness, irresponsibility, drop-out. And you know what? They were correct. All of those qualities applied to me. Children and adults of today who exhibit those traits are described as having an attention deficit disorder, a recognized disease also known as A.D.D. Along with chronic fatigue syndrome, it is a part of the hypoglycemia syndrome, and hypoglycemia is part of the one disease, a degenerated body. Physical and mental fatigue, inability to maintain attention and concentration — all these negative conditions automatically stacked the odds against seeing

51

projects through. Even with $1,500,000 at stake in my 38,000 ounces of silver bullion, I lost the power to concentrate and lost it all, ending up owing my broker a few thousand dollars, plus losing about $150,000 of my own original stake. The same thing happened after I ran $6000 to $53,000 in 90 days in the commodity futures market. The same thing happened every time I played golf. The same thing happened when I was an Officer Candidate in the Army. Oh, I had extenuating reasons all right, but they were all part of the general disease syndrome.

In plain words, I was just plain ol' sick, the result of my ignorance of Mother's laws and how her marvelous machine works. And you know who, besides myself, was at least partially responsible for my ignorance. But you don't have to walk around in the dark. I'm trying to illuminate your path through the morass of misinformation that confronts you daily.

All this talk about "junk food" is valid. The reason most of us don't take it seriously enough is that our knowledge of it is nebulous and not quite complete. If we knew just how food and environmental influences, good and bad, affected our bodies and minds, I think we would take better care of ourselves and enjoy doing it. Moreover, most of us don't really know what is good food and what is junk. We will discuss that too and try to make it easy to understand.

AFTERWORD

I have told you of some indications of above-average capabilities throughout my life. But I have not told you everything. I can cite several more, a few of them truly spectacular. But enough is enough. Notice that I said "indications of above-average capabilities" and not "accomplishments," because my capabilities were in a vacuum, so to speak. They bore no fruit of any significance.

Why were my capabilities sterile? Here again, I hark back to the body-mind relationship, the oneness, the integrity, of that relationship. And you know that I'm emphasizing again how important your physical health is to your overall happiness.

My failures were the result of a sick brain and body which were inherently blessed with talent but which were deprived of energy necessary to exploit the talent.

You will recall that I told you how in almost everything I did, I started out like a champ and ended up like a chump, even when a million-and-a-half dollars was at stake. And I blamed it primarily on the hypoglycemia that dragged on my heels, and mind, all through my days, saying that I always ran out of energy, both mental and physical. That reasoning was for the most part true but not quite complete. All these years another monstrous malady walked hand-in-hand with my hypoglycemia and together they all but ruined my life. In fact, I believe that these two maladies, while not exactly identical, are closely related, the former probably giving rise to the latter.

Only very recently, after I had this book in almost final form, I discovered that I was a victim also of attention deficit disorder, also known as ADD. I had heard of ADD before but never imagined it concerned me in the least. Judging by my numerous frustrating experiences, more accurately failures, I feel that the two monsters had a negatively synergistic effect on each other. In other words, one plus one equaled three. They ganged up on me and put a damper on my development of a healthy productive personality. I always felt a severe lack of healthy aggressiveness and assertiveness. But how can one manifest these qualities when he's running low on fuel?

Inasmuch as it is not one of my purposes to delve into the details of symptoms, I'll just say that ADD keeps its victim for the most part out of touch with reality, forgetful, absent-minded, inattentive, sleepy, and subject to most of the qualities that cause him to be referred to as a ne'er-do-well, a failure, a flop, a goof ball, and odd ball, a misfit. One of its most notable effects is underachievement, and that's my specialty.

More people suffer from ADD than most of us realize, and their numbers are growing. Be informed that children are not the only victims of this terrible condition. Their plight is more obvious only because they're in a stage when their mental and personality development is more conspicuous. The most probable cause of the proliferation of this humbug condition, as far as I can see, is our addiction to our modern way of life, what with all those free radicals bombarding our bodies and brains.

When I read the case histories of some of the ADD patients, I was caught up in a flood of emotion and avoided a flood of liquid tears only by putting the book down for a while and changing the subject in my mind. I saw in their experiences my own childhood, adolescence, adulthood, and indeed my very existence today. Though I had had terrible feelings of inferiority, and even guilt, for having been such a failure, now I know what's causing my shortcomings, and frankly I feel somewhat less responsible for many of those shortcomings. Having a name for the cause helps, because I now have something other than myself to blame, and life is a bit more tolerable.

Alzheimer's disease is another mysterious malady whose "cause is unknown." At least that seems to be the consensus in the medical establishment. Hah! They have always fought tooth-and-toenail against any knowledge that sheds any beneficial light on the cause or cure of any of our physical sufferings. That is, until everybody knows the score. Then they shout it to the world that after intensive research they have finally and heroically found the cause. By the way, arthritis still "has no cause," and is still one of their favorite cash cows, and will always be, as long as we continue to follow the Pied Pipers of America.

Anyway, Alzheimer's also has all the appearances of being closely related to hypoglycemia, certainly of being a product of poor physical health. And several respected specialists have said as much in print.

I should also tell you that I have never learned to type with any degree of efficiency. I absolutely must look at the keyboard or make a million errors. I make many errors anyway, and lose an untold number of manhours finding my place again on the copy and on the keyboard. So you can imagine how long it took me to write this long letter to you and how badly I wanted to write it. I would be embarrassed to tell you how many years I worked on this project. Another reason for my slow progress was that I could never maintain a long working session. After an hour or so, even with a smooth flow of thought at my command, I got fidgety and had to stand up and do something else. This was my attention deficit disorder at work. To you this may appear to be a cop-out, making excuses, but to me it was extenuating, painfully real.

Why should I be telling you about my difficulties? To solicit your sympathy? To alleviate the stigma of my inefficiency? No, not either of them. I'm trying my best to impress on you the resoluteness and earnestness of my efforts, as I have said, "to dissuade you from the mainstream of current medical philosophy onto a path which promises more health and less disease — a lot more and a lot less." Knowing what I had to overcome to get my message to you, knowing what a heavy price I had to pay for the privilege, perhaps you will truly understand how much another human being, a brother, cares about you, your happiness, and that of the entire human family.

I was innately blessed with the brains of a genius, an athletic ability comfortably above average, the strength of a woolyworm, the durability of a marshmallow, the stamina of a cloud, the concentration of a fog, the ambition of an opium addict, and the personality of a shrinking violet. In short, I was and still am a ne'er-do-well.

One of the minor comforts of life is that when one can describe his negative traits in words instead of merely admitting to being a failure, a klutz, or a nerd, he can analyze them and rationalize an infinite number of reasons for them. This wraps a soft cushion around his ego that has already suffered too much. Oh, the blessings of words. But rather than belabor you with more of them, I'll just say that hypoglycemia and ADD did me in. Then I can further blame them on my loving grandfather for having stuffed me with sugar in my tender years. Inasmuch as he is long gone, I don't think he would mind my assigning him some of the blame. After all, he did it lovingly. But unfortunately, lovingness without proper knowledge can sometimes spawn disastrous results.

Now, of course I don't know for a certainty what caused my sad state of affairs, but I can rationalize all I want to whether my facts are correct or not. It doesn't matter as long as I can instill in you the wisdom of being a good steward of your body, the temple of the Holy Spirit, as well as, perhaps more importantly, being a loving steward of the health of your young children, who faithfully depend on you for their future successes in life.

In the military, people earn their Congressional commissions as officers in one of two ways: (1) They go through formal training, either in military schools or, if they are specialists in certain fields, schools in the civilian sector. They go mostly through organized theoretical education. Or (2) they work their way up through the ranks, usually starting out as Recruits, formerly known as Buck Privates. They go through informal self-administered hands-on training, absorbing experience by osmosis, at the cellular level. What they learn is learned "as they go" and requires no further testing by way of working experience. When they earn their commissions, they know which end is up. These seasoned working veterans are known in the military as Mustangs.

Similarly, in the field of health and sickness, some people earn their degrees through formal high-technology education. Their learning is administered by authorities, the powers who determine what's good for the student practitioner and what's to be taught. And what is deemed good for the student is tomes upon tomes of sophisticated study, all leading to the ultimate career: PPD, the Propagation and Preservation of Disease, or what a doctor friend of mine called his cash cow. Now why would anyone want to propagate and preserve disease? Why did Willie Sutton rob banks? Because, he said, that's where the money was. Disease is where the money is. It has value. It is at once the raw material, the product and the merchandise of the medical industry. Most of the training is force-fed, but in the end the rewards of their efforts retroactively render their efforts well worthwhile. The beneficiaries of this prestigious education are trained in their heads, while the cells of their bodies, including their hearts, are often kept in the dark.

In the field of health and sickness, I am a Mustang. To earn this degree I had to learn by and for myself, the hard way. I worked my way up through the ranks in the College of Hard Knocks. CHK has no designated board of regents, professors, or instructors. Students study on their own, conducting their own experiments and research. They learn from their mistakes, their setbacks, and their successes; that is, if they care enough. Or they drop out, forevermore relying on the experts and powers-that-be to govern their lives and determine for them what and how to think.

•

CHAPTER TWO

QUID PRO QUO

Dick Lemming and Belle Trier have stopped in at a sidewalk snack shop. Dick orders a chocolate sundae and Belle, a glass of orange juice. Out of the blue Dick announces, "We sure can thank our lucky stars for all the good doctors we have in this town."

"That's an obvious statement, Dick, but what brought up that thought just now?"

"Well, speaking for myself, I'm not feeling too good these days, and it seems I'm getting sicker more often. My arthritis is getting worse and my heart doesn't feel too good either. It seems my whole body is below par, and that's why I'm so thankful for the doctors. Every time I've needed help they've come through. They seem to know exactly what to give me to make me feel good again. And I guess I should be thankful for all the new high-tech drugs on the market. I guess as long as I can depend on the same super treatment, I won't have to worry too much about old age, except if and when cancer hits me, of course. They say one out of three will get it, so I won't be alone on that. I'll have plenty of company, so I'm not going to worry about it. Besides, we have no control over cancer anyway. And maybe they'll find a cure for it soon."

"You know, Dick, I've always tried to avoid doctors, always thinking Mother Nature would do a better job. So I've gone along with the health nuts. I've eaten health foods, taken vitamins and minerals, gone on cleansing fasts. And you know what? I still keep getting sick. I'm no better off now than I was when I started on this health kick five years ago. What's discouraging is that every time I start something that's supposed to be so great for my health, like fasting, I get sick again. How can all this health stuff be good for you if it keeps making you sick? I hate to admit it but I'm just about ready to give up my glorious ideals and admit you've got the right slant after all. I'm almost convinced that health is the proverbial pot of gold at the far end of the rainbow. I think I'll order me a chocolate sundae too. What's the name of the doctor you like so well?"

Howard Sharpe was moseying by and stopped short. "Whoa, there, Belle. Don't let this poor misinformed buddy of yours throw you off."

Dick responded even before Howard was through talking. "Whadya mean, misinformed? Where does a college freshman dropout get his authority to pass judgment on the knowledge of others?"

"Ho, ho! Listen to Joe College, willya. They're all alike. Give 'em a sheepskin and they immediately become authorities on everything. They've got it all. No more room for any more knowledge. Remember what Alexander Pope said about a little learning being a dangerous thing? Well, Belle, we're seeing it before our very eyes."

Dick could see that Howard was fully resolved to push all the way to the end. "Okay, Sharpie, you teach Belle everything you know and she'll be more confused that ever. Me, I'm gettin' the hell outa here. Belle, I'll try to straighten you out later, if Sharpie doesn't throw you completely off the cliff again." He stands and starts to leave.

Sharpe knew he had Dick on the run and wasn't going to let him get away unscathed. "Hey, Dick, buddy, take it easy. Stick around. There might be something you can learn even from me."

"Not from you, buddy. You been through medical school? When I learn anything it will be from someone with scientific credentials. See ya later, Belle."

Belle felt somewhat sorry for Dick. "Gee, Howard, do you think you hurt his feelings?"

"Probably did. Sorry. But I couldn't let him get away giving you a bum steer. Besides, he's been in my way with you a long time. What ever do you see in the guy, anyway? But never mind that for now. Pull your chair up closer, Belle, and ream out your little ears real good, and put on your best thinking cap, because I'm about to give you a lecture which Joe College wouldn't begin to understand. If you're as smart and open-minded as I know you are, maybe you'll like what I say and maybe like me a little better. And then maybe some day, you and I will have the healthiest kids."

"Oh, stop it, Howard. Don't you know when to quit? I've told you you're not my type."

"Maybe you'll change your mind."

"May bees don't fly in August. You should know that."

"Never mind that for now. Let's get on with the lesson of the day, the lesson of the year, the lesson of your life. Listen, Belle, what I'm going to say is extremely difficult to explain well enough so that the listener will grasp the idea. And I wouldn't try to do it for anyone else. I'm going to try my best to do it this time because I'm trying to make points with you."

"Oh, stop it, Silly."

"Okay. So let's get started. I'm very serious for a change. I'd prefer you didn't stop me to ask questions. Just listen carefully and ask questions later, okay?"

"Okay, Howard, okay. So on with the lecture!"

Howard chose his words very carefully, knowing that at best conveying his thoughts would be difficult. "Two unfortunate and peculiarly confounding conditions in nature lie at the very foundation of man's general inability to understand the workings of his body. I say 'unfortunate' but perhaps I should say it's one of nature's ways of providing man another avenue by which to exercise his superior intellect. These two situations are at once very similar to each other and yet the exact opposites. They make a symmetrical pair. Though the concept is simple it took me a very long time to crystallize it into words. Get to understand it and you will have gained a big edge on sickness and health. Even after you understand it you will probably often find occasions to question its validity. These moments will come when the good doctor gives you a pill and makes you feel like a million again. Being relieved of symptoms makes you feel good and encourages you to continue doing what you're doing to eliminate the symptoms. On the other side of the coin, developing painful symptoms makes you feel miserable and discourages you from doing what you're doing to inherit these symptoms. Or, having done something supposedly great for your health you get severe symptoms anyway. Simple enough."

"Yes, Howard, you know I've experienced all that. Tell me something I don't know."

"Just listen, Belle. Moreover, the relief of symptoms is so gratifying that it feels better than not having symptoms in the first place. Wouldn't it feel better for having stopped sticking yourself with a needle than when you're sitting peacefully watching a colorful sunrise on a spring day? Therein lies the difficulty and therein lies the reason almost all of us appreciate medical treatment to such an unwarranted extent. Again on the other side of the coin, suffering new and more intense symptoms, as you do when you start to fast, makes us so miserable, partly because it's here and now, that we're inclined to put up with all our old chronic symptoms, partly because they have temporarily been relegated to the dim and distant past by man's tendency to ignore the unpleasant until they reappear.

"This pair of related, though opposite, bugaboos are so formidable in their influence on our knowledge of health that if you not only learn them well but doggedly hold fast to the knowledge of their true nature, and also live accordingly, you will have earned for yourself, and perhaps others, a reward earned by very few. Now, what I have told you is simple and obvious, but of what use is it to us who aspire to good health? Well, in plain words, the relief of symptoms, or "getting well" is a siren song. It has lured millions, almost everybody, onto the rocks of ill health. A major deception is involved, because relief of symptoms is not synonymous with getting well."

"Oh, isn't it?"

"No, it isn't. Just bear with me a while so we can get to the other half of the dilemma before we lose the thread. Understanding will come in due time. Suffering symptoms is not synonymous with getting sick."

"Oh, isn't it?"

"No, it isn't. Again, bear with me a while longer, Belle. I'm about to make a few statements which are an affront to the medical establishment and which make up one of the primary pillars of everything I have learned about health."

"Well, hurry then, Howard. I'm all ears!"

"Belle! I asked you to please be quiet. Will you please just listen?"

"Yes, Howard. I'm listening."

"Okay then. (1) Symptoms are not bad; they're good. (2) Symptoms are not disease; they are part of the cure of disease, a healing climax, if they are allowed to fulfill their mission. (3) You cannot expect to pay for your sins, intentional or not, meditated or innocent, without some form of pain; such would be inimical to the wonderful laws of life. (4) It is man's haughty intent to get something for nothing that makes it difficult for him to understand that there is, and should be, a price for everything, good or bad. (5) Medical treatments, when administered to eliminate "disease," are generally not beneficial; they eliminate the real cure, setting the patient up for more real illness in the future as the debilitating agents are allowed to remain, and also to proliferate as a product of the toxic nature of all drugs and other toxic substances inserted into the already suffering body and inhibit the natural functioning of the body.

"Now, the body is endowed with very admirable abilities to perform its normal functions, among which are digestion and assimilation of food, elimination of materials not utilized, and numerous other functions with which we are not concerned at this point. These functions are performed constantly as a matter of routine, gently and without fanfare. But when demands are placed on the body to perform tasks more difficult than routine, it is forced to summon forth means other than routine. These means are commonly called disease or symptoms of disease, which is somewhat correct if loosely defined. But they are more accurately the body's measure to normalize conditions and restore what is called homeostasis. What is sad is that medicine's aim is to remove the symptoms and then declare the patient well, or cured, not considering that the body not only has been prevented from completing its benevolent project but now has an additional toxin or toxins to cope with in the form of the new medicine.

"For example, should you eat food that is heavily contaminated with virulent bacteria or some other harmful substance, your body will probably extract fluids from its own tissues, collect them in your intestines, and carry out the offending substance in the form of diarrhea. And here, sadly, is one of those situations where nature is frustrated by the well-meaning patient, who runs out to the drug store and buys that wonderful pink stuff that coats the stomach and intestines and thereby stops the production of the fluid that is trying to carry the toxins out of the body. Glory be! You have just cured yourself and now feel like a million. Cure enough of these little symptoms and you'll end up with something far worse that diarrhea. Your tissues and organs will be just that much more laden with toxins and perhaps you'll be blessed with an infection, another of Mother's remedies. So you run to the good doctor who will prescribe antibiotics to put those nasty bugs in their place. Hallelujah! The pain is gone. Another victory for medicine and another defeat for mankind. Now the frustrated liver, kidneys, and other organs are hard-pressed to keep the body clean and eventually they themselves will be diseased by the overload of toxins. When the cleaning gang is on the disabled list, who will do their job? Nobody. Then what'll you do? Run back to the doctor? Well, what has he done for you? Oh, he has done something to you, all right, but nothing for you, nothing beneficial, anyway. In other words, medicine has bungled it again. But what's new? Perhaps you should try health for a change."

"Excuse me, Howard, but I wish you wouldn't use me as your example of the misinformed patient. I'm not that misinformed, not anymore anyway."

"Okay, Belle. What I've been telling you is admittedly a bit over-simplified, but it is an example, or microcosm, of how America is killing itself. Most people die prematurely at seventy-five or eighty after ten or fifteen years of miserable health.

"If you still prefer medicine to health, then I haven't explained very well. So far, how does it grab you, Belle? Hey, Belle, now you may speak. I'm asking you a question. Don't you have any comments or questions?"

"Howard, I guess I'm just flabbergasted. And, no, I don't have any questions. I understand pretty well everything you said. Why didn't you explain all this to me before?"

"Well, I didn't want to be presumptuous. I never could get close enough to you to talk about anything, let alone something this controversial and unpopular. But what's to be flabbergasted about? I hope you're not wondering how I could say such stupid things. I still want to know what you think, Belle."

"Howard...," Belle was a bit pensive and uneasy. "Frankly, I never imagined you had it in you to speak so seriously on important matters. I've always seen you as something of a clown. I believe everything you said, and yes, you've made a lot of points with me. You know, you sound just like a doctor."

"Thanks a lot, Belle! But no, thanks."

"Okay, okay. Sorry, Howard. Now, if you don't mind my trying to get more free advice, Doctor..."

"Hey, that's not funny one bit."

"Okay, Howard. I won't ever say that again. Now, how about explaining to me why I always get sick whenever I try to get healthier? That puzzles me no-end. Can you explain it?"

"Yes, I can."

"I knew you could. Now I'm intrigued. And my ears are bigger than ever. Okay, Howard, keep talking. Thy disciple heareth."

"Wish I could, Belle. But remember, I'm on swing shift and I've got to get to the timeclock soon. Some other time?"

"How about tonight?"

"Hey, I told you I'm on swing, and that's 'til midnight. Come to think about it, you're on swing too, aren't you?"

"I mean how about after midnight at my place?"

"Can't do that either. There's a good chance I may have to work over to make some deadlines."

"Then how about lunch tomorrow at my place? I promise you something better than peanut butter-and-jelly."

"You got it, Belle. Gotta go. See ya."

Howard Sharpe made it to Belle's for lunch, and true to her word, she served him much more than peanut butter and jelly sandwiches. But they never made it back that day to discussing her question about her health. They were so engrossed in more personal matters that before they realized it they had to rush again to beat the timeclock. But they met again the next day, and the next, and the weekend. Belle thanked her lucky stars over and over again that she found out before it was too late, what a fine intelligent gentleman Howard Sharpe was.

It was just a matter of time when the couple had to take the bull by the horns and get down to planning their life together. Though Belle had temporarily, but completely, forgotten about her dilemma in health, it eventually had to come up again. And it did.

"Howard, remember you were going to explain to me why I always get sick whenever I try to get healthy, especially when I fast?"

67

"Yes and no. Yes, I remember, and in fact have been waiting to re-introduce the subject as soon as you got ready for it again. You were so busy with more important matters that I figured I'd better wait. And, no, you didn't really get sick when you tried to get well. You began to succeed but always chickened out when you thought you were getting sick."

"Huh?"

"Just sit still and listen, Belle. You're not the only one. Most everybody reacts the same way. First I'll admonish you that you will often find reasons to question the validity of my concepts. After all, symptoms are pain, and pain is bad and unpleasant. It's always been bad since we were babies, and even before. So every time you got a symptom you thought you were sick again, and chickened out. I can't blame you for that. Worse, you thought your noble efforts were making you sick. And that's understandable. Nobody had ever explained to you that your painful and unpleasant symptoms were a healing process started by your conscientious efforts. Had you known the true physiological facts and had been willing to endure the pain and discomfort as the price to be paid for renewed health, you would be a far healthier girl today. As I always say, and will say again, 'Quid pro quo." No rain, no rainbow. There's always a price for everything. Whenever you violate Nature's laws, intentionally, accidentally, neglectfully, or innocently, the price must be paid. And that's just as it should be. Not that I want you to suffer pain. In fact, I would take the bumps for you if I could, though I know I would be robbing you of valuable perspective. Remember this, Belle. In nature there are no rewards and no punishments; only consequences."

"Howard, I have so much faith in everything you say that I just take your statements for granted. So I forgot to ask you, 'Why do you say that painful symptoms are the process of healing?'"

"Good girl! I knew you were going to ask that. Okay, here it is: When the stresses on your body are not excessive and the demands on your cleansing mechanism are not heavy, the adjustments are mild and hardly noticeable. This goes on in your body all the time — when you exhale, when you perspire, and when you go to the bathroom. But when the demands made on your system are too heavy, then more drastic action must be taken to restore homeostasis.

"Say your family get together for a big Thanksgiving dinner and bring a lot of yummy food. After five hours of off-and-on eating, you down three large servings of apple pie ala mode and go home downright stuffed and uncomfortable. Two days later you catch a cold. Now, if you went to the drug store and got one of those wonderful medicines for relief of cold symptoms and used it successfully to relieve the symptoms, you might say that you've gotten rid of your cold. But now there's no cold to do the cleaning job, so the toxins remain in your body and eventually must find some other way to make their escape, and you will probably soon experience some other symptom to do the job, perhaps even another cold. If you persist in knocking off all your symptoms, you could eventually break down with some very serious illness. Basically, in my opinion, this is why there is so much cancer and arthritis around."

"But why must the cleansing process be painful or uncomfortable?"

"Aren't all major adjustments, good or bad, painful or uncomfortable? Shouldn't they be? I'd hate to live in a world where prices didn't have to be paid. Not only that; how can you know you feel good if you don't know when you feel bad? You might say it's part of the laws of balance that are a part of our lives."

"Okay, okay. But why should the symptoms occur mostly when I try to get healthy, like when I try to fast? I say 'try' because I've never followed through, always chickened out because I thought I was getting sick."

"I'll try again to explain. I told you it wasn't easy to understand. It's really simple but somehow the concept is elusive. When you refrain from eating for a while, you relieve your inners from their usual workload and now they can concentrate on doing what they were unable to do while busy digesting and assimilating your food. So now they clean house undisturbed by other requirements. So what happens? Catarrhal discharge, sometimes a fever, itching, headache, a cold, plain old bad feelings, fatigue, somewhat like the fatigue you get when you undertake a big housecleaning. Of all these blessed symptoms, the cold is probably the most effective."

"Wait a minute, Howard. Are you saying that the common cold is one of the processes of healing the body? If you say yes, this is where you may turn me off."

"Again, yes and no. Yes, the cold is a healing process. And no, you're too smart a girl to be turned off, not after I explain a bit more. Tell you what. I notice that you keep old Reader's Digest magazines. See if you still have the issue of October, 1987. Go look. I'll wait."

"I think I have it. Here it is."

"Okay. Turn to page 89. Begin reading here, around the middle of the left column. Go ahead and read it. I'll wait."

Belle reads, her eyes getting noticeably wider. She reads it again. "This is intriguing indeed. I see what you mean. The implication certainly is heavy that you're right."

"I really don't need their corroboration on this. I've known this a long, long time. Many respectable minds are with me on this opinion. Did you read where that German doctor said that people who catch less than one cold a year get cancer six times as often as those who catch one or more colds a year? Remember, this is only an opinion, but it's well founded on statistics."

"Yes, I read that. Isn't it exciting? Howard dear, you're teaching me so many smart things."

"Listen, Belle, you did notice, didn't you, that those statistics were reported by a German doctor and not an American?"

"Of course. Did you expect American doctors or pharmacists to shout it to the world? How naive can you be?"

"Good girl, Belle! Are you getting wise to the world! So you see, if you can believe me, that the common cold is a great blessing. You shouldn't need one, but when you do, be happy to have one. This is when your faith in the system will be sorely tried. You should help it do its job. And that doesn't mean to help it with those high-tech drugs, or any medicine for that matter. Let it do its work and help it by keeping your body clean and not adding any more toxins and stresses. We'll discuss how to do that a little later. Also notice the last paragraph of that article. The author says to respect our colds, that they are part of the genius of nature. I wonder how that was taken by the powers of the medical and pharmaceutical industries."

"But, Howard, how can a cold be good for you when it is caused by germs? I hope you don't think I'm just looking for negative thoughts. They just come up and hit me."

"Super, Belle. I know you're thinking. Keep asking questions and I'll give you the best answers I can. And if I don't know, I'll say so. You might even give me new food for thought. But to answer your question, germs do not cause colds."

"Huh?"

"Neither do fish create the sea. Neither do flies create garbage. You see, as we have said, a cold is a process of cleaning our the body, and so germs come and help out, not because they are kindly critters, but because their work is part of Nature's plan. Their role in the plan is to convert dead organic matter back to dust. 'Dust thou art and to dust shalt thou return.' If nobody did that work we would have billions and billions of carcasses of all kinds piled deep all over this planet. The dear fellows thrive on dead organic matter and feast on it wherever they find it."

"But how come they attack me when I'm not even dead yet?"

"I was afraid you'd ask me that question, because I have to tell you this, Belle: When germs feast on you, you're partly dead. You have dead matter, also known as garbage, in your blood and tissues."

"Where did the garbage come from?"

"The next time before you put something into your mouth, look at it first. You may see your answer there, though I hope not. If you don't, look at somebody else's lunch. You see, young lady, what is not real, live, natural, food cannot be converted to part of your body, and if it's not part of your body, what else can it be?"

"Garbage!"

"You've got it again, Belle! And if it's garbage, what happens to it?"

"Well, it's got to be got rid of somehow. Through a cold?"

"Yes, maybe, or some other form of infection, like sinusitis, boils, acne, or even something like halitosis, body odor, or dandruff. All those undesirable conditions are caused mostly by garbage, sometimes assisted by malnutrition, a deficiency of certain elements needed by our bodies.."

"Hm-m-m-m..."

"Ever notice how an infection almost always heals itself after a while? That's because our little friends have got rid of most of the garbage and run out of food, not only at the point of infection but from other parts of the body as well. You see, as the blood circulates it passes through the infected area and carries garbage there for the germs to dispose of. Neat, isn't it? But if the person with the infection persists in pouring garbage into his body, of course the germs will have a bountiful supply of food and will feast for a longer time. And the person will probably moan, 'I just can't get rid of this blasted infection.' This is how diabetics lose their feet and legs through gangrene. Some of them have so much dead sugar in their bodies that the germs feast until the person dies and is embalmed."

"Howard, I'm downright thrilled to have learned so much valuable information from you. But yet my mind is not quite at ease, and that is because so many millions, probably billions, of sick people are suffering and dying through so much misinformation."

"I must caution you, Belle. These are just our opinions. We may think we have all the answers but we can't say it too directly to other people. That would be like pushing them down their throats. All we should do is offer our opinions to others, and share them unstintingly with those who are receptive, the way I did with you. Remember, Jesus said, 'The poor we will always have with us.' I'm afraid that also applies to the sick, though I wish to God it were not so. Belle, dear, we've talked a lot about sickness. A little

later we'll talk more about health, okay? And after that I'd
like to talk about us."

"Howard, I don't think there's much more to talking
about us. I think we understand each other pretty well now."

"Thank you, Belle." Tears came to Howard's eyes,
something unusual for one so strong.

The developments I have just narrated to you took place
about thirty years ago, in my mind, at least. What has
happened since in the lives of our three characters? Three?
Oh, yes. I had completely forgotten about poor Dick. Sorry
to say that Dick got sicker and sicker and finally succumbed
to cancer. He had been administered chemotherapy and
was gone in two months, having wasted away to 76 pounds.
He was married to a woman similarly oriented to high-tech
medicine and pharmaceuticals. Because he had been
uninsurable when he needed it, he left his family in a horrible
financial position. His widow, formerly a somewhat dignified
lady, now works very hard in a factory. Her daughter, now
18, had dropped out of high school after her junior year
and now works with her mother in the factory. Their
combined wages fortunately are just enough to keep the
family from going under. But should either of them be laid
off, the boy will have to quit school too. Sadly, all we can
do is wish them the best, or at least not too much difficulty.

Belle and Howard, as you probably have expected, have
united into a very harmonious marriage. They have three
lovely children and the entire family is in glowing health,
not only in the physical realm but in the moral and spiritual
as well. Belle left her factory job even before their marriage
and has been a happy and enthusiastic homemaker and
mother. Howard returned to school with money he had
conscientiously begun saving even before he had gotten

close to Belle. He is now Howard Sharpe, N.D. (Doctor of Naturopathy), beloved of the many patients who fill his waiting room. You can easily imagine that Howard extracts considerable happiness from his practice, not only because it provides him and his family a comfortable living but perhaps more because he has the opportunity to help so many people acquire and maintain good health.

You probably have observed that Howard Sharpe and I share a lot of knowledge, or opinions if you prefer. But I did not acquire mine at such an early age as did Howard. I remained in a quandary as I stumbled around in the dark for many years. It was only the Great Life Force that kept me in the ball park. I read, I thought, I experimented, I observed myself and others. All too slowly I gathered new knowledge, albeit tentative at best, for how could I be sure of my thoughts when seemingly very few people on the planet had expressed similar views, as far as I knew. I gained considerable confidence in my views only after the works of some writers had gained my healthy respect with what I considered to be solid truth. My present views were not accepted off the pens of experts merely because they were experts. Some of them gave me food for thought and others merely added to my confidence in what I had learned. Having attained something of great value at a great price, one would naturally want to put it to maximum use, not only for oneself but for others as well. Add to that my compassion for the poor patient being lambasted and promised even more abuse in the uncertain future, and you have a fairly good idea what goes on in my soul as I write this love letter to you, my brothers and sisters.

CHAPTER THREE

MOTHER'S MARVELOUS MACHINE

The fairy tale I have just told you about Howard and Belle Sharpe, as you probably have gathered, was concocted in my head to tune you in to what we'll discuss next. What follows will be somewhat unusual and quite possibly very foreign to you. But it is at the very heart of the general concept of this book. It is my attempt to release you from the shackles of conventional "knowledge" and to share with you what I consider useful insight into how our bodies take care of themselves. You will then be free to examine a broader spectrum of concepts and to more intelligently navigate through life's morass of ideas.

Before we go on, please bear with me a spell while I give vent to my exuberant soul. As I approach this subject, as I behold the wonders of our bountiful world, I get all enthused again. I am compelled to pause for a moment to remind you what a marvelous body you have. This interlude is not intended to lead up to any other point I plan to make. Just thinking about the boundless miracles going on in our bodies is an end unto itself. Knowing, even without fully understanding, only a small fraction of how our bodies operate convinces me without a doubt that a divine entity of infinite power and intelligence is the chief executive officer. An unimaginably infinite number of intricate and delicate operations are going on in our bodies at all times. So faithful is your physiology that only wanton abuse and neglect can throw it off its divine course. If you would contemplate the wonders of our bodies I have given thought to I'm sure you would begin to understand why I chose to write this book. Not to have written it would be an act of ingratitude.

Within my own soul, after decades of living them, I know my opinions to be facts, however different they are and in spite of their lack of popular subscription.

I surmise that many health-oriented entities wonder why so many people still embrace the drug philosophy when the natural approach is so obviously superior and when the former has so obviously and tragically failed us, notwithstanding all its glamorous high-tech accomplishments.

Much can be said for a well rounded and balanced life, and compromise is unfortunately an essential ingredient of such a life. It is not only for a lack of knowledge that mainstream America looks on junk food as its standard dietary fare and on drugs as its standard remedy. To live differently would be too darned inconvenient, depriving, disrupting, and antisocial. Living on the fringes requires strength, self-confidence, and an independent spirit. The typical American not only doesn't know why sprouts are better for his health than the original grain; he couldn't care less. He's having too much fun at the fish fry and at the ball game with his hot dogs and coke. Yes, life is to be lived, and lived with verve. So I think I have a pretty good idea of how people feel about their health and why they live the way they do. And I thoroughly respect their right to use their time, energy, money, and thoughts as they see fit.

Then there are those who feel life is not lived well when the instruments and agents of life are not at their best.

The existence of these two extremes in health philosophy doesn't necessarily mean that it's perfectly okay to drift aimlessly anywhere between the two. To maintain a healthy mind one should at least know where he stands, lest he be buffeted about by the capricious winds of life. My aim here is not to tell you where to stand. All I want for you is a fair chance at obtaining the knowledge necessary to intelligently choose how you want to live. I want you to know who is the best qualified expert to take charge of your health. If you're not an expert yet I will try to make you one, if you care. My fond hope is that enough people do care and that my offerings are worthy of their caring.

"Esprit de corps." No venue can be found more appropriate to this phrase than the bodies of God's creations, including ours. The "spirit of the body" is exemplified and manifested constantly in your body and always will be, as long as your soul remains on this plane. The battle cry is, "One for all and all for one!" A leg is injured and the other one works harder to help its partner and the rest of the body. The entire body compensates to keep all parts in balance. An arm is lacerated and the whole body rallies to its aid, calling on its chemical department to stop the bleeding and to maintain conditions conducive to healing. Even the intelligence department is called in to provide the common sense required for prudent care of the wound.

The body is loaded with toxins and is vulnerable to serious consequences if not soon relieved of the debilitating offenders. So one or more of the numerous body parts serve as overflow points to allow for purging of the entire body. If the body continues to take in toxins, other parts may be called to expedite the overflow. Usually the clean-up project is successful and the body is restored to a state of physiological equilibrium, known as homeostasis. If even more toxins are taken in than the body can purge in a timely manner, more serious symptoms will manifest to relieve the body. It was not only because of a shortcoming of the body that the invasion of toxins was so pronounced, but also of the mind and spirit. The mind and spirit were granted free agency by our Creator, and this is fortunate, else Heaven would be overflowing with undeserving souls.

Now, there are more ways for toxins to enter the body than in junk food. They enter by way of the air we breathe and also through the skin. And apropos of the primary thesis of this book, they enter by way of the doctors' and pharmacists' needles, pills, capsules, and other magic bullets. These latter avenues, along with the rationale and attitudes which foster their use and unbridled proliferation, in my unequivocal opinion, are a major scourge on the health of humankind.

All substances entering the body which are not metabolically useful are poisons, in that they interfere with physiological functions and must be extricated, adding yet more stresses to those of which the body already has too many. Enough of these foreign substances and the stresses they generate, and the body can be loaded with more free radicals than it can successfully manage. (Free radicals will be discussed again later.) The result can be any serious disease, which is really just a symptom of a generally deteriorated body, as well as, more importantly, Mother's avenue by which she disposes of the garbage; in other words, her garbage chute. Just as the expansive beach is made up of individual grains of sand, disease is made up of numerous individual debilitating influences, large and small. This is why I say that every metabolically useless substance is a poison. It does not have to be technically categorized as a poison by a chemist to be one. If it injures the body, it's a poison. By the same reasoning, and in a pragmatic sense, a substance doesn't have to be chemically categorized as a carcinogen to be one. All debilitating substances collectively lead in the direction of cancer, whether cancer is ultimately manifested or not. And as far as our purposes are concerned, cancer is just another symptom of a generally very sick body, no matter how many billions of our dollars "they" pour down the rathole annually to study the deep intricacies of the Big C. "Huh! Just another symptom, you say. The most brilliant minds on this planet have been studying cancer for decades at a cost of billions and still don't understand it, and you say it's just another symptom. How absurd can you be?" Why do you think I call them "Big Medi$in?"

As far as I'm concerned, these prestigious erudite scientists have utterly wasted their energies and abilities, as well as our time, lives, and money, chasing Pandora's butterflies. Even if they catch one, what for? The mystique of cancer is absolutely moot. Even the term "academic" shouldn't be wasted on it. Just a tiny fraction of the wasted billions could be very profitably spent on health education. And you can bet your very last sunflower seed that it would be spent "profitably" if administered by Big Medi$in.

Anyway, who needs to know all the whys and wherefores when you and I can simply treat our bodies with respect and gratitude and glory in the great gifts of life showered upon us? Who needs to know the alloy of our piston rings when we can simply keep our engine clean and supplied with good oil and gasoline?

Now, for your comfort please be advised that we will discuss cancer again when we come to the chapter on Symptoms.

It is not among the purposes of this book to pass judgment on the intellects and morals of our trusted

81

medicine men. They have their own problems and we have ours, many of which are foisted upon us in the form of unnecessarily complicated considerations. Already overloaded, our minds and energies can best be used to resolve our problems in a more pragmatic fashion, or, better, to live positively to the exclusion of excessive problems. After all, we are not pursuing a doctorate in oncology. We simply want to be healthy. And despite the mighty forces working against us, we can if we try.

As long as we're talking about trying, let me say something that should be very obvious but which seems to be a novel idea to most of us: Getting cancer is not a matter of chance. It's a matter of how one has lived. Even where one has tried, ignorance of the law excuses no man, and no woman either. It dismays me to observe people's attitude that cancer is a matter of chance, that we have no say in who is going to be the next victim.

Some of the simplest statements are the truest; conversely, some of the truest are the simplest. But sadly, some of the brilliant minds of today have complicated and convoluted some of our vital concepts to the point where the layman is totally confused, misled, and discouraged. True, there are numerous ramifications to everything, but most of them are incidental to the simple basic condition. Worse, some of them are not even incidental to anything germane to our concerns. While many of them are generally valid, they are unnecessary for, and extraneous to, in fact inimical to, practical understanding and effective solutions.

Let me repeat a statement which I hope will not confuse you with its simplicity: There is only one disease; general degeneration of the body caused by autointoxication, malnutrition and enervation. Let me elaborate. (Here we go de-simplifying already. Sorry.) What are known as diseases are merely symptoms, local expressions of a state of general degeneration. Your body is a wondrous thoroughly integrated orchestra of interdependent parts, all working in intimate cooperation not only with one another but also with all the others as well. There is no such thing as "only" a sick this or a sick that. Should you tell me that you're in perfect health except for your sinusitis, I would tell you that I'm really a handsome fellow except for my face. Common "diseases" such as an arthritic pelvis or cancer of the stomach are not isolated and complete expressions. Before the debilitation can overcome your pelvis or your stomach, the entire body's physiology must be so debilitated that it no longer has the power to regenerate the sick body part. The disease has found its expression through the path of least resistance, wherever in the body that path might be. This "expression" is really an outlet, the body's attempt to purge itself of the foreign substance or substances inimical to its health. If the person cooperates by refraining from absorbing more toxins, the body will succeed in fairly short order. If not, here we have a person who is below par, not "up to snuff," lacking in the "joie de vivre." All sins against Nature must eventually be paid for. One can escape the debt only by escaping the physical realm. And even then, who knows?

Nature has been running this universe, or at least this planet, for eons and eons, and I feel safe in saying she has done a perfect job of it. Any trouble man encounters is of his own making. Man was made perfect and accorded respect by being granted free agency. He can respect his body and soul and remain in perfect health or he can be a sick hedonist. Isn't it great that we have the dignity of choice?

Recently I observed a mother with her three children. She had a unique and interesting characteristic about her

83

facial features and expression. What fascinated me was that every one of her children had inherited the exact unique looks of their cute mama. No blood test would ever be necessary to prove the blood relationship among these four persons. Such perfection of reproduction and yet we have been given the enjoyment of being different from one another, alike and yet individual. Is it any wonder that people-watching is so fascinating?

Do you realize that a person can be cloned from one cell taken from any part of his body, whether that part be his skin, thumbnail, hair, intestine, spleen, or whatever, and that the clone will be an exact duplicate of the original person regardless of the source of that cell? You have heard of hair analysis, by which the chemistry of the entire body is determined. Orthopedists and other physicians can analyze the chemistry of the entire skeleton by taking an "osteogram" of the hand or any other part of the body. Such is the oneness of Mother's Marvelous Machine.

If you have studied any of the biological sciences, you had the privilege of observing how wonderfully put together all living beings are. If you have studied human physiology, you no doubt were awed by the genius which pervades the minute intricacies of our inner works. Physicians, having been extensively exposed to the profound marvels of nature, should know more than the rest of us about the awesome efficiency of the human body and the tender loving care showered on us by Mother. Then why do they even begin to think they do a better job of managing our bodies? It's downright absurd. I must seriously doubt that down deep they really think they do a better job than Mother. Then why do they ridicule us and call us quacks for maintaining a loving respect for Mother, while they pour drugs into our blood? Ever hear of the proverbial golden eggs? To elaborate any more on this question would be to insult your intelligence. Moreover, I can dwell on this subject only so long without crying. The logic of it is so absurd that were it not so outrageously and grossly tragic, as well as costly in terms of life, health, and money, we should pass it off as just a stupid joke.

If all this is so obviously true, why do we flock to these do-gooders by the millions? I really don't have an answer to this puzzle, but I must suspect that the medical schools have a secret course of study in Mass Hypnotism. Or perhaps it's just our human nature to stick with the tried and even untrue until something better comes along. I'm trying to show you that something better.

If you're looking askance at my odd-ball concepts, you should be aware that much of it is subscribed to by many M.D.s who have broken out of their conventional shackles and studied and thought on their own and have had the courage of their convictions. If you feel insecure standing alone or even with a small minority, many health-minded professionals have demonstrated similar philosophies on the subject. Many others are steadily approaching a crystallization of the concepts. But this is nothing new. Our philosophy was well-espoused by respected men and women about a century ago, but that was before money became a god. Consider:

> "*The Greek physician Hippocrates observed that the natural tendency is for sickness to pass and give way to renewed health. Therefore, he reasoned, the role of the physician is to wait upon nature, to care for the sick by diet and hygiene until time has healed them.*"
>
> — William A. Siler in his book,
> "Death by Prescription"

"*What are commonly called diseases are in reality 'cures,'
and the common practice, with drug doctors, of controlling
the symptoms, is like answering the cries and gesticulations
of a drowning man with a knock on the head.*"
— Charles E. Page, M.D.,
1840-1925

"*...disease is a natural process of purification, and should
not be stopped, but aided... Remove the cause and the
effect will cease.*"
— Robert Walker,
1841-1921

"*The medical world has been looking for remedy to cure
disease, notwithstanding the obvious fact that nature needs
no remedy — she only needs an opportunity to exercise
her own prerogative of self-healing.*"
— John H. Tilden, M.D.,
1851-1940

"*The physician who can cure one disease by a knowledge
of its principles may by the same means cure all the
diseases of the human body; for their causes are the same.*"
— Benjamin Rush, M.D.,
signatory to the Declaration of Independence

"*Practically all disease arising in the human organism is
caused originally by the accumulation of these effete waste
and end products of digestion and of tissue changes.*"
— Henry Lindlahr,
very prominent physician
of the early 1900's, 1914

(Of disease:) "*...simply the inability of acute reactions to re-establish homeostasis.*"

— Jonn Matsen, N.D.,
Vancouver, B.C.

"*Disease is nothing else but an attempt on the part of the body to rid itself of morbific matter.*"

— Thomas Sydenham, M.D.,
famed English physician of the 17th century.

"*All sick people carry their own doctor inside themselves. Patients come to us because they are not aware of this truth. The best that we, as doctors, can do is to give that interior doctor the chance to work on the illness.*"

— Albert Schweitzer, M.D.

"*God heals. The doctor takes the fee.*"

— Benjamin Franklin.

Today the doctor gets in the way of God's work and takes a bigger fee than ever.

Until recently, roughly around the advent of the industrial revolution, man had adapted to his natural environment for millions of years and survived pretty well. How can anyone with half-a-brain believe that an abrupt wholesale infusion of unnatural chemicals into our bodies is the way to make and keep us healthy? Let us start thinking for ourselves and stop allowing the money-oriented entities to lead us by the nose to the slaughterhouse. Remember, people major in Marketing in college, and when they get out their avowed aim in life is to separate us from our money by any means necessary and possible.

Adding years to your life is not our primary aim. More important is to add life to your years: pep in your step, hustle in your muscle, zing in your thing — all the things that make up your body and soul. Conversely, I hope you will not die before your official death. Look around you and you will see what I mean by the walking dead. It is foregone that you don't want to be one of them. Questions: Do you expect to be one of them? Are you willing to take charge of your own life and establish a lifestyle which will assure you a long life of quality? How would you achieve your aim of a long and happy life; by placing yourself in the hands of the experts or by taking charge of yourself? If you are not certain yet of the preferred alternative, I will try to give you enough insight to make a choice with conviction.

The state of our health care today (That's what they call it, anyway.) is so intolerable that a crisis is at hand and forcing us to find a solution for ourselves. I'm trying to give you a jump-start toward where I hope you want to be.

The parts of our bodies, including our minds, are designed to be in intimate harmony with one another. They all share the burden of real health care, and so it's one-for-all and all-for-one. Should one of them somehow suffer a misfortune, all the rest will rise to the cause of their fellow. Thus by Nature's design they are all interdependent. They thrive and prosper together, and when they have faithfully completed their work after a hundred years or so of entropy, they all peacefully stop together.

Aside from traumatic injuries, we don't die of any specific cause or causes; we die of our whole life. So when a person dies with — not of — hepatitis, atherosclerosis, or pneumonia, something's not been right. Nature's laws have been violated. Ignorance of the law excuses no man or woman. It is my purpose to show you that you can live in a state of glowing health all your long life until your whole body and soul peacefully exit this plane to enter another. But this is Mother's plan, and if we are to partake of the benefits, we must play by her rules. So we must acknowledge that even in this glorious age of high-technology with its labor-saving miracles, there is no shortcut to add to our quantity or quality of life. There is no panacea, no free lunch. There is only quid pro quo. Thank God for the privilege of winning our prize. Else from whence would come the glory?

The garbage in food, the factors which are not usable by the body and not successfully disposed of, undergoes complex chemical changes, and is deposited in various parts of the body. This garbage is known by different names: arthritis, atherosclerosis, gallstones, kidney stones, bladder stones, tumors of all kinds, arcus senilis, nerve deafness, stirrup calcification in the ears, prostatitis, leathery and sagging skin, etc. The body can and does very effectively dispose of trash but only up to a limit. When we dump poisons into our bodies faster than our bodies can get rid of them, that's when they begin to accumulate and manifest themselves as all those fancy jawbreaker names the doctors give to plain old sick bodies. Only the different specific manifestations allow for the many fancy names and the tomes upon tomes of medical books. But we don't need all that information — just a few simple facts — to be healthy.

If we stop trashing our bodies the arteries will clean themselves, and that is a fact which has been demonstrated many times. Prisoners of war, after months and years of starvation and malnutrition, came back sick in many ways, but their arteries were clean. People who go on long therapeutic fasts emerge with clean arteries.

Your body is somewhat like an automobile in that it produces sludge as a by-product of combustion and has an exhaust system to dispose of waste products. Except that your body has more avenues of exhaust: bowels, bladder, lungs, and skin. If you live as Nature intends you to live, this system will keep you healthy. But in our modern-day ways of living, wherein we overload our bodies with toxins, Nature provides other means of waste disposal. However, these additional measures are not as pleasant as the basic ones. They take the forms of skin lesions, colds, diarrhea, atherosclerosis, wrinkled skin, and all the rest of the so-called diseases.

"Psychosomatic illnesses" is a popular expression, partly because it is a good catch-all and partly because it makes the utterer sound so erudite. But I firmly believe that the term "somatopsychotic" (my own coinage, as far as I know) is far more applicable than "psychosomatic." More mental ills are caused by a sick body than physical ills by a sick mind, notwithstanding the popular opinion to the contrary. Because of the ethereal and nebulous nature of the mind, beliefs and statements concerning it are comparatively difficult to dispute and therefore a convenient haven for those who need an explanation where there is no other available. But then, what would happen to our army of AMA psychiatrists if everyone would put his physical machinery into tiptop shape? Heaven forbid! Be that as it may, numerous mental cases have been corrected with nutritive therapy. On the other hand, how many physical wrecks has psychiatry salvaged? It's not only in the mental realm that body chemistry has proven its superiority over the mental approach to therapy. How about alcoholism, allergies, arthritis, and all the rest of those "mysterious diseases" some of which the medics say have no physical causes? Now there's another convenient catch-all. These educated people who ridicule us who value physical health apparently are not educated enough to know how profoundly the brain is affected by the rest of the body. They take such pride in their intellects but eschew the very factors that would enhance their beloved brains. What makes them think that thought is made up of only the ethereal and that the physiological is not involved in it? Don't they know that thoughts are electrical impulses which must have a physical basis, and that the basis doesn't just happen out of thin air, and that the quality of these impulses varies in accordance with the condition of the body? If this aspect of health, both physical and mental, interests you, I strongly suggest you read "Body, Mind and Sugar," by E.M. Abrahamson, M.D., and A.W. Pezet; "Psychodietetics," by E. Cheraskin, M.D., and W.M. Ringsdorf, Jr., M.D.; and "Mental Health Through Nutrition," by Tom Blaine, Oklahoma State judge.

So strong is my belief in this concept that, lacking any other logical reason, I believe that the insanity of our society today is a direct result of an obviously sick collective mind in turn caused by millions of sick bodies. Because of this I could not conscionably neglect to try to convince President Clinton of its validity. I will reproduce below a letter I wrote to him. It is long but should be of interest to you as a member of our national family.

February 21, 1994
The Honorable William J. Clinton
President of the United States
The White House
Washington, D.C. 20500

Dear Mr. President:

Our people, your people, are in a horrendous state of decay — spiritual, moral mental, physical, financial. And that perhaps is an understatement. We have lost control of ourselves. We commit not only violent crimes but also extreme social and personal indiscretions. Respectable men and women shock their neighbors and families with bizarre and unbelievable acts. Apathy, amorality, and immorality pervade our land. We've made a mockery of the beautiful God-given relationship between the sexes. Our divorce rate is disgraceful, sick, abnormal. Our leaders stand frozen in limbo, at a loss for any rationale, let alone any remedy, to this universally rampant epidemic. In fact, many of them maneuver within, and without, the law for self-serving benefits.

A potential, if only partial, solution to our dilemma is so obvious and so incontrovertible that for many years I have waited for some prominent, recognizable, and authoritative personage to come forth and expound its merits. But alas, none has come forth. So I have wanted to come forth myself. But without credentials what clout do I have? I am just a little boy of a minority ethnic origin, born on a little rock in the middle of the vast Pacific. But somebody's got to do it if we are to avoid sliding all the way into hell. So I can stand around waiting no longer. Though I am only one little member of the club, I am one, a whole one at that, and as such I cry every day as I watch our leaders befuddled by, or disinterested in, a monstrous and destructive juggernaut of a problem which they seem unable or unwilling to resolve.

As the man said (or was it a woman?), I cannot do everything but I can do something. And because I cannot do everything I must do what I can. So this letter to you is an effort to contribute what I hope can be a better world for all. A bit later I will suggest a partial but major solution. Numerous respected and authoritative entities would agree with my concept, and this is why I'm so puzzled by their not speaking out on our dilemma. I will name some of them a bit later.

If my concept is too mundane and unscientific for the consideration of some of our erudite and sophisticated sages let them go grind their axes elsewhere. Don't let them get in our way and please don't let them borrow your stone.

The basis of our irrational behavior and low state of morale is our bankrupt physical health. Yes, our moral bankruptcy is a more immediate cause, but moral, mental, and spiritual sickness is engendered by sick bodies. It is common knowledge that with certain hormones a peaceful, tranquil soul can be transformed into a raving maniac, and conversely a raving maniac can be transformed into a paragon of peace and tranquillity. So there is no reason why the following concepts should be at all novel or controversial. Let me try to explain.

Thoughts and emotions are not merely ethereal will-o-the wisps plucked out of the air. Before one can commit a voluntary act he must first think about it. And of course that thought requires a mind, which needs a brain and nervous system, which in turn must have a body. Let us postulate then, that every act emanates from the body; every voluntary act emanates from the body by way of the brain and the rest of the nervous system. May we postulate also, that a healthy body will beget healthy thoughts and healthy acts, and that a morbid body will beget morbid thoughts and morbid acts? But perhaps this concept is too general and thus far lacking a valid basis. So on the basis that our bodies are a thoroughly orchestrated integration, interdependence, and interaction of all their parts, let us say that one cannot have a healthy brain in a sick body. And it is redundant to say that sick and violent thoughts do not come out of a healthy mind and body.

It is an established fact that refined sugar and other concentrated carbohydrates usurp the B vitamins from the body. It is also established that the B vitamins are absolutely essential to the health of the nervous system, including the brain. A deficiency of these vitamins leaves the brain and other nerves in an unstable state. This is when we have what is called jangled nerves, and jangled nerves are usually the condition which prevails when we plunge a knife into someone else's body.

Why are our children so precocious sexually these days? Why are so many teenagers and preteens having so much sex these days? Refined sugar has been determined to accelerate maturity, and this abnormal acceleration continues until we stop poisoning ourselves. "Oh, but people are keeping younger longer these days. Look at all those young-looking grandmas." Is that so? Take all the drugs and cosmetics away for a week and you'll think you're seeing millions of refugees from a nursing home. Do the growing rates of cancer, arthritis, heart disease, and insanity tell you anything?

About half of our people have low blood sugar, or hypoglycemia, in varying degrees and at various times. Paradoxically, hypoglycemia is caused largely by consuming excessive concentrated sugars. About 30 percent of us have it seriously enough to be diagnosed by the standard tests. If this surprises you or if you don't believe it, it is because Big Medi$in has for many years fought the promulgation of the facts. Don't ask me why; you probably know the rea$on, the same rea$on we spend about a trillion dollars every year just to keep half-well.

Our brains rely exclusively on blood glucose for their energy. Without fuel they go kaput. But perhaps that's not so bad. When they work spasmodically, sputter, misfire, and go out of control, that's when we hear sensational stories on the TV evening news. "Now, how in the world can such a fine gentleman do such an outlandish thing?" I'm trying to tell you how.

Sugar isn't the only poison in our junky diet. I discuss it as an example because it is a major culprit. Errant body chemistry, hypoglycemic or not, wreaks horrible havoc not only on our bodies but also on our brains, minds, and behavior. I know all this first-hand, because I've been plagued by hypoglycemia all my life. I have had to study it in depth because the medical people have withheld the truth from me and everybody else. It has tragically wrecked my life. I almost failed to graduate from high school and flunked out of college. I also had three on-the-job fights in my Civil Service career. You might say that I'm unofficially president of the hypoglycemics of America.

As I have intimated, I am not a recognized expert of any kind, just a very concerned member of the club. I probably lack the professional finesse of literary expression sufficient to impress the educated people who help you run our government. So let me quote just one respected authority on the effects of body chemistry on thoughts and actions. Dr. Robert C. Atkins has authored at least four best sellers and also hosts a radio show which has run more than forty years in New York City. Let's excerpt some of his wisdom:

(Here Dr. Atkins is discussing blood chemistry imbalance due to the standard American diet, also known as the SAD.)

"It's not just your nerves... In fact I have come to the conclusion that in the great majority of cases, it can be all in your diet.

... the large number of people suffering fatigue and anxiety who showed blood sugar findings that were abnormal. And the low carbohydrate diet was able to improve or correct the condition.

The type and quality of carbohydrates, especially sugar, that twentieth-century people eat have been found to play a major role in heart disease, high blood pressure, ulcers, diseases of the colon, allergies, alcoholism, behavior disorders, diabetes, migraine headache, Meniere's syndrome, schizophrenia, and other mental illnesses.

It's time for a revolution in nutrition.

... a housewife who had become edgy and found herself screaming at her children.

Authorities have recited an extremely long list of symptoms due to low blood sugar, all of which I, too, have seen in my practice. The list is headed by fatigue, depression, anxiety, and tension.

... symptoms like headache, blurred vision, mental confusion, incoherent speech, sudden phobias, sometimes even fainting and convulsions.

Or you may go through mood swings, outbursts of temper.

You may be overwhelmed by worry and fear, feel insecure, unable to cope.

Your family may think you are weak-willed, antisocial, shrewish, hostile, hysterical, unpredictable, unstable, flighty, tearful, argumentative.

... National Interview Survey conducted by the U.S. Department of Health, Education, and Welfare showed that of 42,000 households (approximately 134,000 persons) some 66,000 persons reported having hypoglycemia. That's almost one out of two.

We now, for the first time in history, eat most of our carbohydrates in a refined form. Your diet can... completely transform your personality."

Drs. Joseph Nichols, Cecelia Rosenfeld, and Sam E. Roberts have found in their practices a strong correlation between marital discord and malnutrition. Once again, sick minds, sick emotions, sick acts come more from sick bodies than from outside evil forces.

Insane behavior is not our only dilemma. Our so-called "health care system," actually our disease propagation and merchandising system, is no less stupid. But that is another matter which could be resolved if we got the love of money out of the way. Can't the system be truly for health care rather than for the distribution of money? I wish you would ask me about this.

We well know that people are losing control of their minds. The average American consumes about three-fourths of a cup of refined sugar daily. In 1976, 20 years ago, he or she ate 20 pounds of candy, chewed 135 sticks of gum, and downed 450 cans of carbonated drinks. The average twelve-year-old boy drank three cans of soda pop a day. That alone was about three-fourths of a cup of sugar. The statistics should be worse today. Can there be any correlation between our insane behavior and our insane diet?

Dr. Atkins is just one example of the numerous specialists who espouse the body-mind correlation. Just a few more examples:

Carlton Fredericks, Ph.D., author of "Psycho-Nutrition"; Tom R. Blaine, Oklahoma state judge, "Mental Health Through Nutrition"; Drs. E. Cheraskin and W.M. Ringsdorf, Jr., "Psychodietetics"; Linus Pauling, two-time Nobel Prize laureate; Sigmund Freud himself, father of psychoanalysis, who said, "Behind every psychoanalyst stands the man with a syringe."; Abram Hoffer, M.D., pioneer in orthomolecular psychiatry; Carl Pfeiffer, M.D., Director of the Brain Bio Center; F. Curtis Dohan, M.D., Professor of Medicine at the University of Pennsylvania; Henry Turkel, M.D., "New Hope for the Mentally Retarded — Stymied by the F.D.A."; Seale Harris, M.D., eminent pioneer in blood sugar diseases; E.M. Abrahamson, M.D., "Body, Mind and

Sugar"; Stephan Gyland, M.D., specialist in blood sugar diseases; Andrew C. Ivy, M.D., eminent physiologist at the University of Chicago whose career was all but destroyed by Big Medi$in for trying to find a cure for cancer; Nathan Masor, M.D., who proved that psychoanalysis had better move over and make room for "psycho-crinology," defined as treatment of emotional disturbances with hormones and vitamins; Irving Willner, New York City pharmacist.

Can these eminent scientists be right? If so, why have we dragged our feet for many decades while millions are killed, marriages demolished, banks robbed, reputations wrecked, young and old of all four sexes raped, lives ruined? Should we try a new approach involving the body-mind correlation? If not this approach do we have something better? Where is it? Or should we just continue our insanity?

But how do we approach the new approach? How do we legislate healthy attitudes? The same way we legislate morality, I'm afraid. But fortunately legislation is not our only means. Instead we can educate, encourage, and inspire. But how can we do these? With knowledge, by promulgating the truth about health and disease, and by dispelling the gross superstitions and erroneous dogmas peddled by the medical and pharmaceutical industries, not to mention our own F.D.A.

No one relishes the quixotic task of confronting our venerable institutions, but our people are dying unnecessarily and living lives not worth living. They are desperately crying for liberation. This is not a time for twiddling thumbs nor for shrinking back from the powers-that-be. Lives are much too precious to continue to be wasted in deference to an industry that has not only failed us miserably but also has violently opposed any and all health measures attempted by others, thereby perpetuating the business of disease propagation and exploitation. The establishment has taken our health and usurped our wealth by drugging us crazy, half-dead, and full-dead. Now we are bankrupt, surviving only on the trillions of dollars stolen from posterity. It's way past time to stop this immoral thievery.

Our medical people claim to have increased knowledge thirty-or forty-fold in the last thirty years, and yet the rate of cancer has doubled in that time. Other major chronic diseases have also proliferated; in their language, "thrived." Are we sicker because of or in spite of the status quo?

Let me hasten to clarify my views: Certain disciplines of medicine render very beneficial, even lifesaving, services, and I respect and appreciate them profoundly. But by and large medicine has evolved into a self-serving dollar-chasing obsession at the expense of the patient.

Again, how do we approach the new approach? It's not impossible nor should it be unduly difficult, notwithstanding the anticipated opposition to it. I suggest, request, and urge the following action: On the basis of a national crisis, which we certainly do have, create a special commission, ad hoc or preferably permanent, to make a fresh, unbiased, and objective study of our marvelous God-given physiology, its care, and its appropriate remedies, unhampered by the ill-founded medical dogmas now killing us. The fresh knowledge produced must be available to every American. Wholesome ongoing encouragement and inspiration must be a real part of the endeavor. With the movement toward natural health now accelerating, I believe our people are more than ready to be inspired by Operation New Hope (or Operation Renaissance).

A very essential requisite of the commission must be that its membership be thoroughly unbiased. The current powers must not be allowed to control the movement. Remember, they have had their chance and blew it royally. The commission must be staffed with people who have no axes to grind, and that might include a number of qualified laymen.

The cost of the commission could ultimately prove to be virtually nothing when compared to what it has the potential to accomplish given the chance. In fact it should prove to be immensely profitable. The gargantuan cost of health care, now in the hundreds of billions, could be reduced dramatically once we learn what true health care is. (Isn't it downright absurd that health care should be such a major and essential consideration in employment?) And think of the dramatic gains realized when our medical doctors redirect their energies to work with Mother Nature instead of against her. Or am I being too naive again? If so, many nature-oriented doctors, long unexploited and persecuted, stand ready to do the job.

In trying to get your attention, Mr. President, I dare to dream of changes which would not only free ourselves from the negative forces of corruption but also reclaim the wholesomeness which enriched our lives before we got too big for our britches.

To the extent that the abundant literature is correct, the people of Hunza in the Himalayas have no crime and no police force. With conscientious effort they protect themselves from the rambunctious influences of the developed world. They nurture their land and respect the virtues of healthy living. Ninety- and hundred-year-old young men father children and play polo. They do not hunger for alcohol or other drugs.

If we could complement our Yankee (and Southern) ingenuity with the practical intelligence of Hunzaland, we just might come up with a true-life Shangri-la. If they can do it, we can do it. Or is this still another naive pipe dream? What do you think, Mr. President?

Inasmuch as this is an open letter to you, Mr. President, and because you have asked our participation in the affairs of our nation, I am sending copies of it over the breadth of our land to some of the largest media. A hundred thinking brains should produce more and better perspective than my hypoglycemic one. Please allow me to appropriate a small portion of this letter for the purpose of addressing any and all who read it. To you readers I say: If you like the substance of what you read here, please discuss it with others, as many as possible. Help make this a successful national crusade. Especially to those who are well qualified by having gained solid knowledge on the subject, I appeal to you to jump in with both feet and join in on this effort to bring our brothers and sisters back into life. Please do whatever you can to enhance the project. This may be our last chance before America bites the dust.

May I thank you now for your active and spirited participation? May God bless our efforts in whatever we do — because what we are doing is right.

> Yours for a happier America,
> Bertram J. Wong (signed)
> 509 East Fort Street
> Manchester, TN 37355

P.S. The U.S. of A., the world's richest nation, ranks behind (worse than) 21 developed nations in infant mortality statistics. Every twelve minutes one of our precious women dies of breast cancer. Rome's aburnin'. Time's awastin'. Let's toss the ol' fiddle and git with the fire hose — or somethin'.

That was my letter to the President. I sent copies of it to the editors of the 141 largest newspapers and health-oriented magazines in the land and also to the ABC, NBC, and CBS television networks. I enclosed a cover letter with each copy asking the editors and managers to help in the crusade, or what I had hoped would be a crusade.

Now, I'll have to admit I did no better in my crusade than Don Quixote did in his. I received one very brief form letter from one of the President's assistants. That was it. Not a single editor responded to me. As you can see, I put a lot of effort into that long letter and also spent a bundle of time looking up addresses and mailing about 150 copies and cover letters. But that's how life goes sometimes. Crusades were never meant to be a frolic around the Maypole and the crusader often finds himself standing alone with no one to dance with. But the fat lady has not yet begun to sing. Anyway, I hope the letter gave you new ideas to contemplate.

I've been saying, "Don't they know" this and "Don't they know" that. You probably already know that those were rhetorical questions, that all the time I had my tongue in my cheek. To be very candid with you, I think Big Medi$in does know all that stuff, but if they don't, it's because they don't want to know. And who can blame them? If you were making a killing on the ignorance of your customers, would you try to educate them? Wouldn't you try to create a false need to keep them coming back to you? Well, maybe you wouldn't, but some people do such things.

I do not relish reflecting on the character of the American doctor. Most doctors are fine people but have been sucked into the mainstream of the industry. If I'm going to write about medicine and health, I'm going to have to write about medicine and health, and "tell it like it is." I must give you a perspective without which my theses would be almost meaningless for having been grossly watered down. In short, I want you to be healthy and I don't want you to spend your life savings trying to and failing to be healthy. But to be healthy without losing your nest egg you must know the pertinent facts as you go about your endeavors. "You shall know the truth and the truth shall set you free."

Do not try to change the sea. Just set your own sail. But to set it right it helps to know the tide.

Whether or not you're willing to pay the price for health, I want you to have a few statistics which might bear on your attitude on the question. Your body is heroically faithful in trying to keep you functioning and feeling well. But don't let that lull you into complacency. Research at Tulane University revealed that of a large number of people who felt well and thought they had no problems, ten percent had asymptomatic ailments, problems which did not show yet but which would probably blossom in the future into major illnesses. These people exemplify the type who are seemingly healthy, usually feeling good, but actually in a way unfortunate in having a physiology lacking in varying degrees the natural propensity for occasionally purging the body by means of minor symptoms. Of some of them might be said some day, "He was never sick a day in his life, and then out of the blue, this." Out of 100,700 people who felt healthy six had cancer without knowing it.

If you would like some really practical and valuable education, go visit a nursing home every once in a while, and while there keep saying to yourself, "There ain't no such thing as a free lunch." Remember, time marches on, and you'll have plenty of time to become one of these if you do not pay the price of discipline while you can.

Of the men examined for military service in World War I, 21.3 percent failed to qualify. For World War II, 41 percent failed. The Korean War, 52 percent. The Berlin Crisis in 1961, 71 percent. Of the disqualifications, 60 percent were physical and 40 percent mental and emotional. Average age was 22. Poor children! Of 200 autopsies performed on soldiers killed in the Korean War, 77 percent had hardening of the arteries. In muscular fitness tests given to American children through high school age, 57 percent failed to measure up. Of European children of the same ages, 8 to 9.5 percent failed. Did you notice the unmistakable trend in the military statistics? America is overfed, undernourished, underactive, and overpoisoned.

What are the major contributors to the shameful state of our nation's health? (1) agricultural practices, (2) dietary habits, (3) non-food factors: smoking, alcohol, other drugs, slothfulness, environment, cosmetics, industrial products, etc., and (4) government politics as influenced by the medical and pharmaceutical conspiracy. So in matters of health do not look for help to Big Government or Big Medi$in. Doctors don't deal in health; they deal in disease. Without disease they're dead. With universal health they're dead. With sickness they thrive. And do they thrive! Need another picture? Never mind.

If the specter of cancer, arthritis, the rocking chair, or a full set of false teeth in a glass of water, doesn't concern you, think of your children and the rest of posterity. You've got the ball.

Where does all that yucky stuff come from when you have a cold or a boil? Would you rather it stayed in your body and didn't come out to bother you? Your pharmacist can take care of that. Why do you have to feel so yucky when you're sick? What should you expect for having violated Mother's rules? Besides, what do you think would happen if you felt good all the time regardless of your state of health? Yes, you're right. You'd sing your merry way through a short life and then die a premature death.

The cleaner you are inside, the more efficiently will your glands and organs function, which means the more efficiently will they keep your body clean, which means the more readily will they produce symptoms when they are needed to purge your body.

It's okay to feel bad now and then. It's analogous to feeling pooped when you clean your big house. It's Mother's way of letting you know the state of your health, and she favors you with symptoms to restore your well-being. Then you feel good and energetic all over again. But you can have this advantage only if you give Mother a chance to help you. Remember, you're a free agent, free to live as you please. But don't expect to reap a harvest you did not sow, nor to escape the consequences of your misdeeds, including your negligences and your hedonism. You make your own bed.

In general, do not try to heal your symptoms unless you simultaneously help them out by cleansing and nourishing

106

your whole body. If you need help, seek it from a practitioner who respects Mother, observes her rules, and enlists her help. A good bet would be a naturopathic or homeopathic physician, a chiropractor, or other wholistically oriented practitioner. Sorrowfully I must say that the osteopathic physicians as a group knuckled under to Big Medi$in a few decades ago and now push drugs seemingly as readily as their new partners. In exchange, they are granted AMA eligibility and the AMA has stopped persecuting them. There's nothing now to persecute for anyway, because the osteopaths have repented and are now well-behaved little boys. I hasten to salute those few who have refused to prostitute themselves.

Should you feel I'm overly biased for the nature boys and against the Biggies, you should know that just a few years ago the Chiropractic Association won a 13-year legal suit against the AMA, who were found guilty of unfair practices. They had infiltrated the chiropractic ranks and undermined them from the inside for many years. This comes under the heading of medical ethics, an oxymoron, no less.

I have repeatedly observed cases, very pathetic cases, where the symptoms were relieved but the patient suffered more as a result. A neighbor of mine got the shingles, the adult form of chicken pox. "Fortunately," as most observers would see it, the medical-pharmaceutical industry had developed a very effective and expensive drug which nips the disease in the bud by drying up the external lesions and preventing new ones from erupting. If you've ever had the shingles you would probably say, "Oh, what a blessing." But I thoroughly believe the drug to be a horrible curse, from what I have seen of its blessings. My neighbor told me that the lesions dried up pretty smartly but that he

107

experienced the worst pain and suffering of his entire life, despite having had two bypass operations, the first one a triple and the second a quintuple. He said he couldn't possibly describe the pain and that it was like the worst possible toothache throughout his entire body. Worse, it seemed to last forever, and nothing would relieve it. He added, "You still couldn't possibly know what I'm talking about." Another friend suffered the same treatment. Her little $89 vial of magic bullets dried up her lesions also, but, as I see it, locked in whatever toxins Mother had intended to relieve her of. (Please don't tell me not to end a sentence with a preposition, because that is the kind of affectation up with which I will not put, and neither did ol' Winnie Churchill.) She also suffered indescribable long-lasting pain in the form of a terrible "toothache" throughout her body. There is yet another horrible case of the shingles I know of, the patient in fact being related to me by marriage. His case is so persistent, having gone on for several years, that he was on the Forty-Eight Hours program on national television. This case has all the earmarks of being incurable. I can only hope that impression is wrong.

Judging by my own experience, I feel the shingles were never nearly this bad in days gone by. Consider my case I contracted in 1977. When I had developed six lesions I sought relief from a doctor. (That was before I wised up and before, thank God, that miracle drug was developed for shingles.) He told me there was nothing in this world he could do for me to stop the progress of the disease. "There is only one thing you can do with your shingles; let them run their course and put up with the pain for another couple weeks, at least, like everyone else. And you may as well expect six or eight more sores to come up." I didn't quite buy his stuff. I went home and put myself on a moderate fast, eating only "clean" foods, fruits and vegetables, and only enough to sustain my energy. Additionally I took a pretty good complement of organic vitamins and minerals, including heavy dosages of vitamins C and E. For good measure, several times daily I rubbed vitamin E into my six lesions after scratching them open with my fingernails. (Remember, germs don't bother me. We'll talk about them again soon.) I reasoned that if any more bad stuff wanted to come out it still had six open doors. Well, what happened? The sores stopped hurting and gradually dried up. No more erupted. The original six were it. Period. Best, no internal pain developed. I had helped Mother heal my body of an ailment which "had to run its course," and did it by making my whole body healthier. After all, there is only one disease.

The lymphatic system, for some reason, is comparatively seldom discussed in print or in conversation. But it is an extremely essential part of your body, being the main pillar of your immune system and several times the size of your blood system. The lymph nodes, like the tonsils and adenoids, serve as collection points for toxins, and it is here that the system ambushes toxins and renders them harmless. But one disadvantage the lymph system has is that, unlike the blood system, it has no pump to circulate its contents through the body. It needs help and with that help it does a super job for you, acting as a drainage canal for purging toxins. The help it needs is muscular exercise, and this is a major reason exercise is so valuable. In a stationary body, lymph does not circulate and thus cannot do its job. This is one reason why being bed-ridden compounds a patient's illness. It has been said that with an efficient lymphatic system it is almost impossible to be sick. That may be a bit of an exaggeration but it makes a good point. Later, in the section on exercise, we will discuss a very effective exercise to enhance your lymphatic system.

After what I would surmise to be millions of years of wondering what made his body sick, man has gradually narrowed down his search to more and more specific causes. He has blamed evil spirits, the gods, curses, the weather, bacteria, viruses, overwork, psychosomatic effects, junk food, and whatever else his mind could suspect. Some of these causes were no doubt valid. Now modern science has come up with and identified a factor which is at once general and specific — general because it is involved in every case, and specific because it is at the very tip of the analysis. It is the immediate cause of the trouble, whatever the trouble might be. The original causes may be thrown out when the study gets down to pragmatic seriousness. Let's call this thing the common factor in all degenerative disease. It has been named the "free radical." Remember this name, because it will be much more involved in our discussion, if not directly, between the lines, and because it causes so much misery to all but those few souls who have taken full responsibility for their health. These people minimize the quantities of free radicals in their bodies and of course enjoy better health. For convenience we're going to use the term "free radical" pretty loosely to identify various aspects of disease, as we flit from one aspect to another.

What is a free radical? It has been defined as an oxygen molecule with an unpaired electron. This lonely electron, reactive in nature and thus in desperate search of a mate, makes its host molecule very unstable, which in turn makes its immediate environment very unstable, which in turn jeopardizes the stability of the entire body.

How do free radicals come into being? In answering I could wax very scientific and delve into chemical equations, but that would not be practical. So let's be pragmatic and simplify, sticking with language germane to our primary objective, which is to understand how your body works. So, again, how do we get free radicals? Through stresses, which may be arbitrarily categorized as dietary, emotional, environmental, traumatic, and a few others. These stresses translate into internal damage wherein physical and chemical changes take place and attack your cells. When cells die they become carcasses and collectively become garbage, which in your body is inimical to the intended metabolism, and so we call them poisons, or toxins.

Observe this scenario: A freight ship has been at sea for over a year on a very tight schedule and no shore leave has been given the crew. Now all the freight has been off-loaded, the scheduled pickups made, and the mission is now completed. The ship finally docks at a peaceful little port named Happytown to replenish provisions. The crew are given shore leave. Each sailor is loaded with money and get-up-and-go. He also has an urgent need to bring his emotional life back into equilibrium. Can peaceful little Happytown remain peaceful while these free radicals are on the loose? Is it unreasonable to expect the town's stability to be jeopardized? The sailors are having a ball getting into and causing all kinds of mischief. A few marriages and other romances have been jeopardized by the presence of these swash-buckling, free-wheeling men. Other crimes are committed. Some of the crew even refuse to return to the ship as scheduled. The small local police force is unable to control them or get them to leave. If Happytown suffers too much for too long, and if it is not to be completely ruined, the National Guard or some other authoritative power will have to be called in to get rid of the free radicals.

The analogous situation described above should give you a fairly good idea of the deleterious unrest which goes on in your body when free radicals are created and allowed to rampage.

Let's find a common example of how free radicals are generated. Take a grain of wheat. It consists of the endosperm, the starchy and largest component; the germ, the rich reproductive component; and the bran, the fibrous outer covering. The grain doesn't become real food until it is moistened with body fluids and its components mixed together. Then it goes through the physiological processes and is converted into blood and body tissues. But man, for commercial advantages, has made it a standard practice to disintegrate the wheat grain by separating the three components and using only the endosperm, the starchy body, as a major food product. The germ and the bran have comparatively little commercial value, being used mostly for feeding livestock and to a lesser degree by health-conscious people. Now when the endosperm, in the form of white flour products, is eaten and ready to be converted to life-giving food, it finds itself alone without its partners, the germ and the bran. It cannot participate in the intended chemical reaction to nourish the body, because the other required ingredients have not been brought along to the jobsite. So what does the white flour do? Mostly nothing. This is a major reason we are so nervous and unstable. It's a relatively simple carbohydrate easily converted to sugar, energy, and fat. Now, to avoid unnecessary chemical talk, let's be very practical and just say that the white flour, or whatever it has now become, is a free radical. Since it is no longer teamed up with its original partners, it is now extraneous material, or in plain words, garbage. And it putrefies like any other garbage. The resulting products are extraneous to body functions and therefore amount to plain old trash, or toxins, to be, if possible, expelled from the body by the normal processes of defecation, urination, respiration, and perspiration. Whatever part of it is not thus expelled, being free, engages in various kinds of troublemaking. It also serves as good food for the cesspool-type germs in your body, which in turn have their own way of making trouble. (If you're interested, these germs are named Escherichia coli, the same E. coli that killed several children who ate contaminated hamburgers a few years ago.) Eventually most of the remaining white flour products are expelled from your body by various means such as colds, sinusitis, acne, eczema, vomiting, diarrhea, infected wounds, athlete's foot, and an endless variety of other infections. Unfortunately, when your body is overloaded with trash, your cleansing organs are included in the overload and thus lose some of their efficiency. Now the toxins are not so readily expelled and are trapped in your body, and this is when your real troubles begin. Your body is diseased and the disease manifests itself in what the medical industry refers to as various diseases but which are merely local symptoms of the one disease. Whichever site of the body is the most vulnerable at the moment, plus the chemistry of the toxin, determines where the trouble will show itself. It may be arthritis, hypoglycemia, stomach ulcers, heart disease, alcoholism, allergies, or, when your liver, gallbladder, and the other organs finally cannot handle the load, ultimately cancer. "Gee, this Joe Blow sure knows a lot about the mysterious disease which our educated scientists still can't figure out."

I will continue to tell you as we go along what I think I learned in the College of Hard Knocks and in post graduate work. In due time we will discuss how we can minimize the harmful effects of free radicals. But I may as well tell you now of a well written little booklet by Zane Baranowski which explains the subject admirably. It's entitled *Free Radicals*. I found it in a health food store, gratis. If you can acquire one of these the same way, good. But if not, you should be able to find a similar treatise on the subject by the same author in your library. Mr. Baranowski explains that free radicals are the result of stress, in this case meaning any adverse effect in the body, the four types of which are chemical stress, emotional stress, physical trauma, and infection. The last two you know about. You know you don't want to break a leg or get into an auto crash. So we can leave that to you.

Right now I must take you on a side trip on a subject that's off the mainstream of health but one I must address, because it affects so many people, especially women, traumatically. The subject is step ladders and stools or chairs used for reaching high places. More tragic accidents involve ladders, stools, and chairs than most of us expect. And sadly, many of these accidents happen to women, and I hate so much to see women injured. The spirit of Women's Lib notwithstanding, women in general tend to be unfamiliar with the physical laws of ladder safety. The big bad word in climbing accidents is overreaching. When the climber reaches too far to one side, the longitudinal axis of his or her body is no longer vertical, but slanted. The slanted thrust of the body-weight now pushes the ladder or stool in the opposite direction. If the overreach is excessive enough, down goes the climber in a most sudden, awkward, and uncontrolled manner, with sometimes catastrophic results. No need to explain how badly hurt one can be in such a fall. The body's center of gravity also plays an important part in the loss of balance. When it gets too far past the support point, in this case the closer legs of the ladder or whatever the climber is standing on, gravity is allowed to assert itself and the climber suddenly and unexpectedly loses altitude. Whatever safety precautions apply to ladders and stools apply also to whatever else one might use to gain altitude. So, especially ladies, please, oh please, be careful and cognizant of the dangers whenever you stand on something. Remember not to overreach. Better to get down and move your support. Thank you!

You also know you don't want infections. But if you're smart you know that what you really don't want is a toxic condition of your body that requires elimination by an infection. Yes, that's a bit difficult to accept, and I understand. But ride along with me a while, just to humor me, okay? Anyway, you won't get many infections if you keep your inners clean. We will discuss how, a bit later. The unwanted toxic condition is caused by undesirable substances taken into the body by way of the mouth, the nose, the lungs, and the skin. It results also from the internal combustion products of physical exercise, as well as from indigestion and poor intestinal health.

Simply put, free radicals undermine your health by damaging and destroying your cells. When your cells die your tissues die, and when your tissues die part of you dies, and all of you that dies is garbage and further adds to your toxic overload. The poor get poorer if they don't know, or don't care, how to build up assets. The sick get sicker if they don't know, or don't care, how to build up health. That is why you see so many corpses walking around among us. Just a little more dying, and...kaput.

When the cells of the skin are attacked by free radicals, they collapse, leak their fluid, and dry up. Now we have that unwelcome phenomenon we call wrinkling. (Sorry.)

Free radicals attack any part of the body that is vulnerable. Some attack the synovial (lubricating) fluid in the skeletal joints. When enough of the lipid (fat) cells are gone, there goes your lubrication, and now you have one of those popular items of conversation — arthritis, bursitis, and their related maladies, all localized symptoms of that one disease, a generally sick body.

You probably have sensed that when we talk about wrinkling and arthritis, we're talking about another unwelcome phenomenon — aging. All adverse conditions of the body are aging. In fact that's the sole function of free radicals — to age the body and mind. But that doesn't have to happen before we have lived our vigorous one hundred years. Remember that it's not age that makes us old men and women; it's aging.

Notice that I did not talk about your aging. That's because you are not going to let much of that happen to you before your time. You're going to help me make my long letter to you worthwhile.

Let's not fret too much about those free radicals, but that doesn't mean they're not bad. Of course they're very bad, but we can decrease our fear of them and live a more tranquil life if we take charge of ourselves, keep them out of our bodies, and destroy the ones we already have. Fortunately, and characteristically, Mother provides a means to do all that. It's called antioxidants, because they minimize oxidation, or decay, or putrefaction. They're also called free radical scavengers, obviously because they destroy free radicals and minimize their effects. Mother provides antioxidants not only in the body as a natural product of metabolism, but also as a natural part of other aspects of nature, especially food. But let's save this subject for a more thorough study in a later discussion. But remember the word antioxidant, because it's a big deal and you will hear about it more often in the years to come.

AN AMAZING DISCOVERY. I had always known, at least as long as I have been cognizant of the rampant medical shenanigans, that modern allopathic medicine has strayed many country miles from the teachings of its father Hippocrates. But because I have been in the comparatively tiny minority who bemoan the departure, I have often wondered whether I have been too harsh in my appraisal of modern attitude and practice. Then, lo and behold, I recently came upon a direct quotation of Hippocrates himself which has caused me to respect the old fellow even more than I had in the past. Let me tell you what he said:

" When disease has attained the crisis or when a crisis has just passed, do not disturb the patient with innovations in treatment either by the administration of drug or by giving stimulants. Let them be."

The medical philosophy of the Father of Medicine is further discussed in "Growing and Using the Healing Herbs," by Gaea and Shandor Weiss. According to the authors, Hippocrates recognized, and differentiated between, two approaches to illness: (1) elimination of the symptoms and (2) restoration of health. He thus drew a line between the medical practitioners of today: the allopathic, or conventional, doctors on the one hand and on the other, most of the alternative practitioners — the symptomatic "healers" and the wholistic "healers." I placed quotation marks around "healers" because no man or woman has ever healed anybody. He or she merely tries to set up conditions which make the body receptive to Mother's healing. Some of these "healers" deserve some of the credit for helping Mother and some deserve blame for making the patient sicker. Unfortunately the blameworthy ones too often receive undeserved credit and money while the more creditable workers are scoffed at and called "quacks" by the real quacks. Do you think Hippocrates would feel honored to be called the father of modern medicine?

You can easily infer from Hippocrates's statement above that he considered a symptom to be a healing event which should not be aborted by anyone but the patient himself, and the only proper way to do that is to restore the whole body and thus eliminate the need for the continuation of the healing crisis, or symptoms. When a crisis is aborted with drugs the healing is aborted and though the patient feels better the illness remains and in fact is made worse, not only because the cause or causes have not been addressed, but also because more toxins have been added to an overstressed body.

You can also easily gather from almost every word in this book that I agree wholeheartedly with Hippocrates. And I am profoundly honored that Hippocrates posthumously agrees with me. I have espoused these theories for about four decades, mildly at first, then with increasing conviction as I progressed through the years in the College of Hard Knocks. My education was given a boost when I noticed who had an axe to grind while basing his practice on erroneous concepts.

My experience in the crucible of sickness and health has taught me an added concept I have not seen expressed by anyone but which I am certain Hippocrates also espoused. For the sake of emphasis let me repeat the concept expressed above, because it is one of the basic theses of this book:

" *When a crisis is aborted the healing is aborted, and though the patient feels better the illness remains and in fact is made worse, not only because the cause or causes have not been addressed, but also because more toxins have been added to an overstressed body.*"

Please bear with me while we go back in time for a spell. (I've said something similar already but this easily warrants repetition.) For untold eons man ate nothing but pure, unprocessed, foods direct from Mother. And he apparently adapted fairly well, given that he is still with us. Reasonably good health probably was his usual state. As he grew in experience and intelligence he progressively "improved on

Nature" and probably fared fairly well for a few thousand years, because his body, with its provident life force, was able to accommodate the excessive stresses imposed on it by these improvements in lifestyle. But about a century-and-a-half ago modern man had "arrived" and was now a very experienced and enlightened being. He began his wholesale improvement of all aspects of his life, his food included. A hundred-fifty years is but a twinkle of a star, if that long, where natural adaptation is concerned, and man has been very hard put to cope with his new lifestyle. In fact he is now faring miserably. Whereas in the past all of his food was natural and simple, and its unassimilated factors were naturally and routinely purged by his body's wondrous machinery, today's vastly "improved" foods contain so much non-food, so much material completely foreign, alien, to his body that his physiology is no longer the slick-running machine it used to be. How could it be, when it's fed mostly contaminated fuel, it's improperly and inadequately lubricated, and when it does run it runs on a cold engine, a condition conducive to low efficiency and excessive wear and tear? It is also highly inefficient in purging the products of combustion from its system, more succinctly the materials left over as by-products of inefficient metabolism.

Let's get back to the practitioner who purports to heal us by aborting Mother's natural healing processes. It is a rare event when an allopathic physician sends his patient out of his office without some drug in his system, his pocket, her purse, or in the form of a prescription. That drug is poison. "Whoa there! How in the world can you say a drug is poison when you don't even know what it is?" I know what it is. It's poison. Any dictionary will tell you that poison is any substance which is debilitating to the body. Any substance you put into your body that is not assimilated as building material is poison. I hasten to say it has not always been so. In yesteryear, or yestereon, when the byproducts of metabolism were easily purged from the body in natural processes by means of more-than-adequate natural faculties, these byproducts by-and-large did not remain in the body long enough to putrefy and intoxicate the body. But today in our high-tech society, where a much greater proportion of what goes into your mouth and lungs and through your skin is inorganic and cannot possibly be assimilated into your tissues, the byproducts are voluminous and your organs and glands have a marginal ability, at best, to cope with them. In most people a huge backlog is waiting in line to be discharged. They wait so long that they become permanent and integral fixtures of the body. To compound the problem, the very organs and glands responsible for the purification and purging are themselves affected by the impurities, much as an overloaded filter and pump might be. Their very tissues are impregnated with debilitating materials which render the organs and glands less efficient in fulfilling a task much more demanding than intended by Nature. So, then every bit of trash piled into the system, in addition to being useless, adds to the backlog of garbage sitting there with little hope of being dumped out before stinking up its environment and taking the body down yet another notch toward some eventual serious illness. And don't forget that while this is going on, the poor liver, kidneys, pancreas, gallbladder, and their teammates are under increasing strain to do their jobs. Eventually some of them utterly fail and go kaput. Surprising? Disappointing? On the contrary, it's a great wonder that our heroic bodies perform as well and last as long as they do, given the abuse they're subjected to. And that abuse includes the tons of drugs stuffed into our bodies by the medical and pharmaceutical industries. But that's not all. While awaiting disposal in the huge trashpile, some of these drugs, in addition to having stopped the healing process, also engage in unnatural and undesirable chemical reactions sometimes, almost always, detrimental to the body.

Are drugs poisonous? Gimme a break!

If you're shaking your head and wondering how I dare utter such nonsense in the face of the abundant conventional wisdom, consider the following:

Is conventional wisdom getting results? Are the incidences of cancer and heart disease on the decline? Are nursing homes cutting their rates and going out of business by the thousands for lack of business? Are we spending less and less on health care? (Health care? Don't we mean disease propagation?) Are children getting cancer these days at a later age?

Conventional wisdom until a couple decades ago was, "Athletes should never lift weights. They'll make you muscle-bound, slow, and clumsy." But there were some dissenters. Bob Hoffman, editor of "Strength and Health" magazine, at least as far back as the early thirties, fervently urged athletes to train with weights for better performance. He dared to say unlikely things in the face of conventional wisdom. His upstart "irresponsible banter" is now conventional wisdom.

Conventional wisdom from time immemorial until about thirty years ago was, "NEVER apply water to a burn injury. Exclude air immediately by coating the burned area with oily medications." Once when extremely hot roofing tar splashed on my hand I ran to the dispensary for help and headed straight for the wash basin. "Doc" jumped up and restrained me. "NEVER apply water to a burn," he said. "But, Doc, this blasted heat is digging in deeper and deeper. I gotta stop it from cooking me." "Hey, Bert, you a doctor? I went to school eight years and spent thousands to learn medicine. I know what's good for your burn." Well, the heat did continue to eat away at my flesh and also caused intense pain. I landed in the hospital with a cooked hand and stayed nine days. By now you know that immersing a burn in ice water as soon as possible is the current conventional wisdom. Again, as Will Rogers said, "A lot of folks knows a lot of things that ain't so."

Even up to this moment, I understand, the American architectural standard calls for a height of 31 inches for a bathroom lavatory. Sometime in the fifties Cornell University conducted a comprehensive study on kitchen efficiency. They determined, by measuring oxygen consumption, that for a five-foot-three woman the most efficient height for her hands was 38 inches above the floor. That's two inches above the standard 36-inch-high kitchen counter, and so we know that our kitchen designers are pretty much in the ball park as far as the fairly short woman is concerned, although her domesticated six-foot husband would find more comfort at a higher work surface. Now, in what significant aspect is the bathroom lavatory different enough to warrant a much lower top surface? Being five inches lower than a kitchen counter, it's obviously about five inches too low for the five-foot-three woman. So can it be nearly comfortable for her six-foot husband? And when he reaches down into the wash basin, it's lower yet. I am confident that the only reason everybody seems to accept the stupid standard height of the bathroom lavatory is that it's conventional wisdom and that he's never bothered to question it. I am also confident that if all bathroom lavatory countertops were built 36 inches high, everybody would like them better, even though some people wouldn't notice the difference. I know a man, somewhat short, who shampoos in his kitchen sink every day. Could height have something to do with it? I installed my bathroom lavatory countertops 36 inches high and am happy for it. Conventional wisdom certainly dies hard, sometimes at great cost.

I could go on and on and tell you about Cristoforo Colombo's defiance of conventional wisdom. I could tell you about Louis Pasteur and how he contradicted even his own conventional wisdom about germs shortly before he died. But I've allotted conventional wisdom more space than it deserves. But consider one more thing: Is conventional wisdom sometimes powered by that green stuff?

There are reactive minds and there are creative minds. There are blind followers and there are thinkers.

We self-righteously and smugly ridicule the beliefs of the less-developed peoples of our world, referring to them as superstitious. Hah! What about our own big time superstitions? We do have some of them.

For example, we think we're in good health until the forces of evil attack us from the outside. "The flu bug is going around." "Johnny's got cancer. Boy, you never know who's going to get it next."

These victims are innocent bystanders who just happen to get hit by random attacks of bad luck. We seem never to think that they are guilty of contributory negligence.

Not only are we superstitious. We're irresponsible.

By now you probably have correctly sensed that I don't place much value in discussing specific symptoms, that I prefer to depend on general health to keep the body free of specific symptoms. But following this I will devote some space to discuss a few popular and common "diseases," for two reasons: (1) to try to dispel some prevailing concepts of disease and (2) that such discussion will tend to cast additional perspective on the general concepts we have been discussing.

CHAPTER FOUR

SOME COMMON SYMPTOMS

INTRODUCTION

I will condescend to discussing specific symptoms only because they are a vehicle wherein the average reader, hopefully not you, is still absorbed. They should serve as a comfortable bridge over which I hope to lead you from where you are to where I would like you to be.

All symptoms are brought on by unfavorable living conditions: lack of exercise, slothfulness, physical and emotional stresses, dietary indiscretions, and, perhaps to a lesser degree, environmental conditions.

To be sure you and I will be on the same frequency as we discuss symptoms, though at the risk of being overly repetitive and pushy, let me repeat one of the essential theses of this whole discussion: There is only one disease, a general degeneration of the body. What are popularly referred to as diseases are merely symptoms, local expressions of disease, Mother's healing measures to restore health, or homeostasis, to the body. To "cure" a symptom is to frustrate Mother by aborting her healing process.

If you have a problem differentiating between disease and symptoms, let me try to help. Disease is an unhealthy condition of the body which cries out for relief. Mother provides that relief by producing a symptom. The need for the symptom is unfortunate but the symptom itself is a remedial, restorative, corrective event, a blessing from Mother.

125

Say your indiscreet dietary habits have resulted in indigestion and consequent piling up of decaying food in your stomach, duodenum, and intestines. So you become nauseated and throw up. The toxemia from the decaying material is disease. The nausea and vomiting are symptoms, benevolent symptoms. Would you prefer to feel sick and vomit or would you prefer to keep the putrefying stuff to yourself? If you prefer the latter, go see your conventional doctor or your pharmacist. They are eager to cure you. Otherwise be thankful for your symptoms and don't try to "cure" them.

"All violations of Mother's laws, wanton or innocent, must be paid for." The payment may be made in many small installments, one big one, pay-as-you-go or an accumulation of repeated debits in the form of capital charges and compound interest, and perhaps bankruptcy. The misery of physical symptoms are one of the conditions and part of the price of payment.

If I had to violate, I would opt for pay-as-you-go. Sadly, the huge majority of debtors habitually place stop-orders on their payment checks, in the form of drugs of all kinds. They consequently develop increasingly larger debit balances which eventually must be paid. There is no free lunch. Then there are some violators who lack the resources to make even small payments and who therefore eventually go bankrupt under the huge load of accumulated violations charges. Of these people you have heard it said, "...and he was never sick a day in his life."

For hopefully obvious reasons I do not intend to devote too much paper to discussing relief of symptoms. First, I do not believe in stop-payments on legitimate obligations, and even if I did, such a discussion would distract from the primary concepts I'm trying to convey to you.

126

Should it occur to you that I seem to be contradicting myself by suggesting remedies for certain specific symptoms, notice also that suggestions I offer are ones that are not commonly found in the hundreds of other health books. If I did not share them with you, for whatever they're worth, you might be deprived of knowledge which could be of some value to you. Moreover, this is my way of keeping on the good side of the reader who might still be obsessed with symptoms.

"If you don't want the M.D. to drug me, what else can I do? Just stay sick?"

No, you don't have to stay sick. If your symptoms are comparatively minor irritations, and if you observe most of Mother's laws, especially with the additional guidance I offer you in this book, you should find yourself in pretty good shape in a few days or weeks, because with a little help Mother still takes care of you. Haven't you noticed that minor symptoms which are not part of chronic diseases like arthritis and atherosclerosis always run their course and vanish on their own? If you must go to a doctor, try to find one who loves Mother. His medicines will be health-giving substances rather than injurious drugs. Whatever doctor you go to, let's hope he doesn't drug you, however legal that drug might be. If he does, you can help minimize the damage by living the kind of life advocated here and in other health-oriented books and articles.

A special note:

You don't have to point out to me that I have been overly simplistic and idealistic in my approach to prevention and treatment of disease. I really don't mean to be that biased and dogmatic. Trouble is, the medical industry has such a strong grip on the public mind that I have had to drive pretty hard in order to pull you out of their grip long enough to get hold of your ear. Despite all I have said about our M.D.s, by and large they personally are good people and, given our attitude toward health and disease and the consequent personal neglect of our own health, M.D.s provide a beneficial service. But I'm trying to alter our attitude to a point where we will allow Mother to do her job, because she does it right.

We will discuss M.D.s in better perspective when we get into the chapter on Big Medi$in.

The following discussions of symptoms, collectively, should contribute to your general understanding of the message I'm trying to share with you.

MALIGNED and MISTREATED MICROBES

Are you superstitious about germs? (What kind of stupid question is that?) Do you believe germs wear black hats and attack healthy innocent people? If you do, sorry, you're superstitious. What makes superstition is somebody's belief that another doesn't buy, and I don't buy the germ theory. But when you believe something, then it's knowledge or faith. So perhaps to you I'm superstitious for appreciating germs. Good. Now we have a basis for discussion.

"Germs are persona non grata and cause disease." If there ever was a concept that has been dogmatically espoused not only by the medical establishment but also by the populace at large, that concept is it. There's not the slightest doubt that germs cause disease. Even if the statement is not often expressed verbatim, the concept is alluded to millions of times daily. We are preoccupied with protecting ourselves against germs. Numerous TV commercials and printed advertisements cater to this fear, and of course foster it also. Coincidentally and conveniently, this fear supports

128

huge industries the world over. So why am I so quixotic as to try to upset such a huge applecart? No, I'm not trying to do such a thing. But I am trying to do what I can to share facts which I believe could provide perspective to the quality of your life.

Let's for the moment open up our minds and allow their contents some elbow room so that we may move them around a little to see if we can find a better arrangement of the facts.

As we did just a while back, let's assume some germs have invaded your "stomach" and have caused a nasty infection, what is popularly called intestinal flu. Too bad, because you were feeling so well and having a ball when the bug bit you. And now you're miserable and weak, feeling absolutely puny and effete. Then after a few days of misery you begin to feel better, then better still, until you feel your jolly old self again.

Why were you so fortunate as to have those invaders retreat when they had you down and defenseless? Why didn't the nasty varmints go for the kill when they could have? Before the attack you were well and strong enough to repel the invaders, but somehow they got to you. Then when you were completely defenseless against the rampaging invaders, when they were on a roll, they withdrew and abandoned their hard-won territory.

There seems to be something illogical about this story. But come to think about it, the same funny thing happens every time you get an infection of any kind. Can you explain this poor example of military strategy? Okay, then. Let me try.

Your body, to begin with, was loaded with more toxins than it could tolerate, and so, in Nature's wisdom, the germs came to help you clean house. They consumed the excessive dead organic material and changed its composition. In the

129

meantime your body took advantage of this new scene of activity and brought toxins from other areas to this collection point for disposal. Then, on cue, it provided a river of fluids to wash the waste material out. You had a benevolent case of diarrhea. The excessive toxins had been disposed of and the germs had completed their task and their services were no longer needed. They left. Shortly after, you felt hunkydory again.

Does that explanation make sense to you? The medics don't buy it. Why should they? They're not stupid. They may be something else but they're not stupid. But I buy it, because it's true. And it will remain true until I hear a better one. It's the same old story. Mother knows best.

If you have a problem with the theories of a rank amateur, contemplate the following:

Even the revered Louis Pasteur, by consensus Mr. Germ himself, said before he died that, "the resistance of the individual is more important than germs in the causation of disease."

> "If I could live my life over again I would devote it to proving that germs seek their natural habitat — diseased tissue — rather than being the cause of diseased tissue."
> — Rudolph Virchow,
> "father of cellular pathology"

> "...and the greatest of all delusions is the Germ Theory, and the consequent introduction of serum therapy, with its various antitoxins."
> — Thomas Morgan, M.D.,
> in "Medical Delusions"

> "...they (microbes) are not the primary and fundamental cause of disease. ...the condition of the host is the primary

factor. Bacteria are so important to life that we cannot survive without them. Germs don't cause disease — disease creates an environment favorable to the proliferation of germs."

— Alex Burton, M.D.,
eminent Australian professional hygienist

"Germs do not cause disease. Nature never surrounded her children with enemies. It is the individual himself who makes disease possible in his own body because of poor living habits. Do mosquitoes make the water stagnant, or does stagnant water attract the mosquitoes? ...Germs are friends and scavengers attracted by disease, rather than enemies causing disease. ...As the internal environment is, so will be the attraction for any specific microorganism..."

— Robert R. Gross, M.D.,
professional hygienist, New York

"The germ theory has suited man's ego quite well. Most of us prefer to believe that the illnesses we suffer are the result of external forces — just as we would rather blame bad luck for our failures. ...as though we are in no way to blame for the medical catastrophes that befall us."

— Drs. E. Cheraskin and W.M. Ringsdorf, Jr.,
in their book "Psychodietetics"

If we can accept the theory set forth above, it is sadly ludicrous that people in general have such a superstitious fear of germs. "I need after-shave lotion so my face won't fester." "When massaging your scalp great care must be observed to use only the balls of your fingertips and not your nails, lest you puncture your scalp and invite infection."

131

"Be sure to replace your germ-laden toothbrush at least once a month." And so on, and so on, and so on.......

You realize, of course, that precautions such as those cited above are uttered by the superstitious among us, and perhaps rightly so, because they are vulnerable to the discomfort of the work of microbes. We who are enlightened and live prudently are exempt from threat of infections. But should we get an infection, we view it in realistic perspective.

Get hold of the Reader's Digest issue of February, 1995, page 61. Please do it; it'll be worth the effort, I promise. If you think that article is a satirical joke, you're not alone. I thought so too, until I read on. It's downright pathetic and at the same time unintentionally extremely comical. To see how afraid this high-tech scientist is of ordinary germs in ordinary everyday situations makes you wonder if he's serious. Sadly, he is. For example, his and his family's toothbrushes must be kept at least six feet from the commode, because the Escherichia coli bacteria are flung that far in the spray that is created whenever the toilet is flushed. And also importantly, he flushes the toilet with his elbow. Says he, "If you keep your toothbrush within six feet of it, you're basically brushing your teeth with toilet water." Every few days, he advises, disinfect your faucets, refrigerator handles, and shelves. Enough, already! I didn't know whether to laugh or cry, but I didn't have a choice. I did both. Isn't it pathetic that man has come to such a relationship with God's creatures? I said "Enough, already!" Okay!

Now, I'm not saying germs have nothing to do with infections. I'll even say that germs cause infections, if we can define infection as a cleaning action. Granted, infections are accompanied by pain, but remember, you have violated Mother's laws of health and are responsible for the pain.

"In nature there are no rewards and no punishments; only consequences."

— Found in a fortune cookie

So don't go blaming your woes on my little friends who have come to help you out. After all, it wasn't they who stuffed your face with junk.

What is superstition is the belief that germs are the malevolent agents of disease in otherwise perfectly healthy bodies and that infections are unfortunate events. Whereas germs instead are benevolent workers who come to drain the debilitating factors which would otherwise bring on more serious misery in the future. The intended result of the germs' cleansing action is a reasonably healthy body condition, or what is called homeostasis.

Just so you won't think I have always been a healthy specimen who doesn't speak from experience, let me tell you what happened one day when I was twenty years old. I was visiting with one of my aunts at her home when she said, "It's too bad."

"What's too bad?" I asked.

She hesitated, then said, "Oh, never mind. It's just too bad."

"Hey, let's not go with this half-way stuff, eh? What's too bad?"

"Well...well, you're always blowing your nose! It's disgusting." She had finally got it out. "Uncle feels the same way. Ever notice that he never gets close to you? He likes you but is afraid of your germs."

133

Can you imagine how humiliating it was for me, a twenty-year-old, to be called disgusting, to have someone afraid of my germs? And yet I guess they were not unreasonable. For as long as I can remember I had carried a wet handkerchief in my back pocket against a cold wet butt. If you want to talk about a case of chronic hay fever, a cold, sinusitis, or whatever it was, this was one. Throughout the week my handkerchiefs turned gray from constant handling, and every Saturday afternoon I boiled, bleached, washed, ironed, and folded about twenty handkerchiefs, starting the new week with a fresh supply of snow-white hankies and ending it again with ugly gray ones. Oh, what misery it was also to always have a sore red nose. You can understand why I have compassion for those poor puny people with red noses. Well, those years of sniffling and nose blowing ended abruptly in 1954, when I had had enough of ill health and attacked my problem in earnest, mostly with the help of Prevention magazine, then a somewhat new publication. I had had it with handkerchiefs. From then until now I have never regularly carried a hanky. In Tennessee, only on Sundays I sometimes carry one to church if it's cold, just in case I get a dew-drop nose from the winter weather. Other than that, no more handkerchiefs, no more cold wet butt. Oh, it's so nice to have a warm dry one.

As I have implied, I was once a very puny young man. I had colds, hay fever, sinusitis, prostatitis, boils, headaches, flu, all kinds of infections. In me the bugs had found Paradise. In my early youth I was underweight, round shouldered, and usually appeared to be looking for money on the ground. "Bert! Straighten up! Lift your head up!" I was tired of hearing all that stuff, but what was there to feel good about? But all of that ended in 1954, when I took the bull by the horns as explained above. The results I experienced were so dramatic and impressive that I'm still a health nut today. At that early stage of my education I had not made any assessment of the popular germ theory, nor had I formulated any of my own. Only after many years of study and experience did I gradually zero in on what I know, or believe, today.

I haven't had any kind of flu since 1954. I guess I had had my share of it by then. In the forty years since, I have needed colds to help me out only four times, and each occurrence had an explainable cause. None of them came in the course of my prudent living. But it's okay to need a few symptoms now and then. That's what they're for. There's some merit to the saying "Better to wear out than to rust out." Once my eyes were swollen from springtime allergy. Whereas I had rid myself of all allergies in Hawaii, springtime allergy has troubled me on the mainland. Anyway, the pharmacist said I had an infection in my eyes. I didn't think I did but maybe he was right. I've also had a few dental infections, but other than those I have been completely free from infections of any kind. I have very little fear of germs, as I consider them my friends.

Another friend, the late Paul Bragg, an eminently popular health lecturer, used to say to his audiences, "If any of you work in a laboratory and have access to bacterial cultures, bring me a culture when you come for tomorrow night's lecture. I don't care what kind of bug it is. I'll do with it whatever you want me to. I'll eat it, inhale it, rub it in my eyes, stick it my ear. Germs don't bother me, because I'm clean. I don't have trash in my body for them to feed on." Like everyone else, I suppose, I thought Mr. Bragg was an appropriately named windbag and was bluffing. But now I'm sure he was sincere, because I now also do not fear the little dears. Of course I'm not as daring as Mr. Bragg was, but I am reasonably invulnerable to infection. I got this way by keeping my body clean, shunning junk food for the most part and trying to a reasonable extent, to observe Mother's laws.

Why are we always fighting Mother's creatures? Kill, kill, kill! "Smush that nasty old bug!" "Kill that damned snake!" He may be just a harmless garden snake but kill him anyway. "All snakes are no damned good." Isn't it a sad situation? The world is such a wonderful place given to all of us by God as our home. All other animals are at peace with us. It is we who are at war with them.

In His Sixth Commandment God said, "Thou shalt not kill." He didn't say, "Thou shalt not kill other people." Nor "Thou shalt not murder," though some modern translators have arbitrarily mistranslated the Word that way. God said, "Thou shalt not kill." Period. The longer I live, the more I respect the Sixth Commandment.

"If germs make me feel so bad, how can you say they're helping me?" Well, there's no free lunch. There's only quid pro quo. If you violate Mother's laws, you're entitled to know it, and pain is your signal. Without pain you'd soon kill yourself. And without germs, what would you do with all your junk? But you wouldn't have to worry about that very long, because Digger O'Dell would soon take care of you.

If you don't want roaches running wild in your kitchen, don't leave soiled dishes on your countertop all night. If you don't want germs in your body, don't stuff junk into your body. But if they do come, don't kill them. Keep your body clean and you can quit fearing germs and start living in harmony with them. Except for considerations of esthetics you can just about forget about sanitation.

I have submitted that germs are our friends. Even if you disagree, does it not make more sense to live healthfully and coexist in harmony with them than to fight them? We know without doubt that by fighting them we merely challenge them to bolster their defenses and develop more resistant and potent strains of themselves, ultimately to become deadly enemies and cause misery for us.

Which brings us to another critical subject: Antibiotics. T.C. Fry of Life Science, a wholistically oriented organization, is right when he says, "If a million people do a stupid thing, it's still a stupid thing." When 260 million people do a stupid thing, it's till a stupid thing. Ironically, the very sciences which develop knowledge in what kills life are in the forefront of knowledge of what builds resistance to adversity and how biological organisms adapt and develop into durable strains. And yet, look what they have done to our world.

Well, what have they done to our world? And who are "they?" They are almost everybody: doctors, patients, pharmacists, the FDA, and everybody else who doesn't care about our world, who doesn't bear the responsibility for its welfare. But the "who" is not important now. It's too late for that. What is important is that we as a whole society become more discriminating in the use of antibiotics. It's very discouraging, I realize, what with the monster of a problem we now face, but what choice do we have but to try? Yes, this sounds awfully naive, but somebody's got to say something. And moreover, we all have got to do something about our attitudes toward our little friends. We simply cannot leave our fate in the hands of the people we have trusted to skipper our ship. If you don't know what the problem is, man and the microbes have been waging war for half-a-century and the battles have become more torrid. Man has been the aggressor and the bugs the defenders, but the bugs have done very well, because God is on their side. And that is because we have turned against God. As an example of what's happening, the organisms which "cause" meningitis and respiratory infections can now thumb their noses at tetracycline, heretofore one of the dependable standbys for these ailments. Not only that; tetracycline is now a favorite food of yeasts. Oh, what have we done!

So we thought we had tuberculosis licked? I hope you know it has come back with a vengeance. And now we're waiting for Big Medi$in to heroically find a silver bullet again. Oh, what a bunch of clowns we have been!

I have alluded to the stupidity of the antibiotic movement. This is not Monday morning quarterbacking, but as far back as World War II, when the use of antibiotics flourished on the military fronts, this flunked-out student of bacteriology could see what troubles lay ahead. After the war these drugs were prescribed with seeming abandon for almost every complaint from a patient, even though it was known that they were ineffective against viruses, which are supposed to be the cause of the common cold. They were prescribed as "preventive therapy" even when no ailment existed. I recall complaining vehemently about this recklessness. I also recall declining to fill my doctors' stupid prescriptions for the stupid drugs. But all I could do about this huge problem was to feel hopeless and blow my steam, just as I'm doing now.

The other side of this coin is not pretty either. While we have helped our chosen enemy to build himself up into a powerful army, we have coddled ourselves into becoming little wimps, hiding behind the skirts of our antibiotics. Our immune systems have been terribly compromised. If you're not worried now about our plight, in a few years you will share my worries.

There is really nothing too terribly wrong with antibiotics, just as there is really nothing too terribly wrong with fire. It is the irresponsible, reckless, wanton, rampant use of it that has us now holding a tiger by his tail, and I'm afraid the prognosis ain't so hot.

Let us summarize what our medical industries, the Unholy Trinity, are doing for us; more accurately, doing to us.

(1) They frustrate Mother's attempt to clean house. When an infection is stopped, the purging process is aborted and the toxins remain in the body to continue jeopardizing its health with the potential to cause more serious mischief at another time and in another area of the body.

(2) They challenge the microbes to develop more resistant strains of themselves, thereby holding the potential to bring into being incurable diseases. Notice that we have some of those already? Unless man is able to maintain his one-upmanship against the germs, more incurables will be coming along. We have made enemies of our friends.

(3) They kill microbes indiscriminately, the good with the bad. Moreover, they have turned good ones into bad ones. There is no telling how many millions of patients have had their intestinal flora destroyed by antibiotics, never to know as long as they live why they never feel well, why they are now constipated, why they now often have gas and diarrhea, why their digestion and assimilation are so subpar. Poor innocent victims.

(4) They rob our bodies of the incentive to build up their own defenses, causing us to be more and more dependent on them. We are now a far different animal from what we were in the pre-antibiotic days.

(5) They are forcing our friends to act like enemies. In the escalating war between us, I'm afraid that man's ability to continue to develop new and more potent antibiotics is limited, or at least questionable. But our "enemies," with the Great Life Force behind them, will probably meet every challenge of our scientists and ultimately overcome every new drug thrown in their path.

If you want more perspective on this tiger whose tail we are hanging onto, see the Reader's Digest issue of March, 1995, page 78. But it's not joyful reading, and don't say I didn't warn you. Yes, we live in troubled times. But what should one expect when man gets too big for his britches?

I don't know. Granted, we need antibiotics. We're in too deep and now have no choice but to swim. Ecologists would probably say we should have, in the first place, allowed Nature to do her own job and not have interfered with the law of survival of the fittest. All we can do now is to use our wisdom and restraint and, provided Big Medi$in doesn't drag us into deeper water, perhaps bring the war back into equilibrium.

THE COMMON COLD

How do we fight the common cold? Please don't! Let's not repeat the epitaph "Killed by friendly fire."

For generations the common cold has been maligned, demeaned, derogated, detested, and despised, all to our detriment.

Then how should we treat the common cold? With respect, honor, and gratitude. For it faithfully comes to your rescue when you have failed in the care of your body, more accurately, when you have abused your body. Whether the abuse is wanton and perpetrated through a lack of responsibility or whether through a lack of knowledge, if you would like to be healthier by means of increased perspective, read on and contemplate our discussion. Just for the time being, ignore what you have been taught by the Establishment and keep an open and flexible mind.

Incidentally, what I say here about the function of the cold applies also to just about all other symptoms of our bodies, what are popularly termed "diseases" but which are merely various outlets for toxins in a generally sick body. I have harped on this concept before and will harp on it again.

Let's get back to the cold. It would be far better if you hadn't accumulated so much trash in your body, but you have, and it's fortunate that you have the ability to toss it out. The ability to "get sick" varies between individuals. Those "fortunate" healthy persons who "have never been sick a day in their lives" often surprise their friends and families by suddenly getting cancer or a heart attack. Do you recall the research we reported in the chapter Quid Pro Quo which revealed that people who catch fewer colds get more cancer?

Do not try to get rid of your benevolent cold. Above all, do not even think about antibiotics. For one thing, the cold germ is a virus, and antibiotics don't kill viruses. Shun laxatives; they severely jeopardize your homeostasis. Don't be taken in by TV commercials hawking Contac, Tylenol, and all the other nature fighters. "Cure" enough colds, dry up enough sinuses, stop enough perspiration, and you'll be a front-running candidate for something much more serious than the benevolent cold.

To help your cold finish its job you should minimize the addition of more junk to your system and maximize, or hasten, the purging process. Eat only wholesome, clean, live, natural food, mostly fresh raw fruits and vegetables. If

141

you're conscientious enough go on a fresh fruit and vegetable juice fast. This is a way of giving your body some degree of rest while still providing nourishment. Take a good measure of antioxidants: like vitamins A, C, and E; selenium; and pycnogenol, an exciting and comparatively new discovery in America, though it has been extensively used in other countries for quite a few years. We'll get back into pycnogenol when we discuss internal cleanliness and nourishment. Get in as much rest as you conveniently can. Try to get enough sleep and maintain a tranquil spirit. Here's the reasoning behind the beneficial effects of rest: Energy is required to support body movement, emotional stresses, and especially muscular effort. Moreover, stresses add more toxins to your already overloaded system, tending to exacerbate your cold. Energy is required also for digesting food. When you are working, playing, or otherwise expending energy, and when you still have undigested food in your system, your body cannot very efficiently accomplish much else, since there is only so much energy at its disposal.

If these conditions accompany a cold, the cold is more or less held in limbo and will take more time to cleanse your body. But spared the responsibility of dealing with stresses and of digesting food, your body has more energy for cleaning house. And when your system is clean, your organs and glands, being part of the system, are clean too and in better condition to help you create more energy. So you can see that rest is not only the cessation of the expenditure of energy; it is also a condition in which the body is allowed to rejuvenate itself.

One of the more effective measures employed to shorten the need for a cold is the enema, or in its more thorough form, the colonic irrigation. Edgar Casey, the famed Sleeping

Prophet, is reported to have said that one good colonic irrigation is as effective as ten days of fasting.

Why have our best medical minds in countless generations and despite intensive efforts failed to cure the common cold? Don't you know that a cure would bring billions of dollars into the pockets of somebody? Instead all they have done has been to stop the symptoms and frustrate Mother's attempts to purge the body of trash, while building a foundation for more serious illness in the future, and in fact have without doubt caused untold misery to humanity. Anyway, a cold is not a thing; it is a profound and powerful process ordained by our Creator for the upkeep of His temple. Should anyone succeed in finding a cure for the common cold, woe be unto the human race.

I think it's pretty naive to assume that germs exist to harass other beings. To the best of my judgment their basic function is to return dead bodies to the earth, from whence they came. They do this by consuming dead organic matter, and never attack healthy blood or tissue. When they go to work on you, you're at least slightly dead. Sorry. This means you have excessive dead matter in your body and your little friends have been assigned to help you clean house. If allowed to finish their work they'll get you in better shape than you were in before you "caught" the cold.

Let's nail this thing down "real good." Our disdain of colds and most other symptoms is every bit as erroneous as our ancestors' belief that our world is flat. But I fondly hope that within the next generation or two we will come to appreciate our symptoms as the beneficent healing work of Mother Nature and loving gifts of our Father Creator.

Yes, I realize how presumptuous and condescending this makes me appear, but if it were my mission to hang rose-colored glasses on your nose, I should never have bothered to write this letter to you. Amen.

THE BIG "C"

I will not accord as much space and honor to cancer as most people think it warrants, because it is not the big heavy enigma most people have been taught to believe it to be. If that sounds a bit flippant and outrageously presumptuous to you, be informed that a goodly number of qualified researchers share my view. If they don't promulgate their (our) concept as loudly as the mainstream entities do theirs, perhaps it's because they aren't as intent on grinding their axes, or because they don't have a huge hard-driving business organization behind them to further their fortunes.

You may or may not have heard of Dr. Max Gerson. But you very probably have heard of Dr. Albert Schweitzer, often referred to, while he was still with us, as the greatest living human being. He called Max Gerson the greatest genius in medical history. In three separate episodes, years apart, Dr. Schweitzer, himself an eminent physician, enlisted the medical expertise of Dr. Gerson for puzzling illnesses of his daughter, his wife, and himself. Dr. Gerson came through in every case, the last one being the "curing" of Dr. Schweitzer's cancer at age 75. Gerson himself said that he merely helped Nature do the curing. Schweitzer lived fruitfully until the age of 90.

While we have the light on Dr. Gerson, and before I give you his explanation of cancer, I should tell just a little about this highly intelligent man. He came to America from Austria in the early forties and to my knowledge never joined the AMA gang. Because of his different and threatening medical philosophy, Big Medi$in with the solid help of the U.S. Congress persecuted him mercilessly for the rest of his life. The shenanigans involved are in themselves a shameful, poignant, and criminal story. He certainly was not a typical M.D., in my opinion far above joining the herd. He "cured" numerous "terminal" cases of cancer, and for many years maintained a standing invitation to his medical critics to visit his clinic and observe his methods of treatment. That invitation still stands today at the clinic operated by his daughter Charlotte Gerson in Bonita, California. Of course, in all these years none has responded to the invitation. In opposing and persecuting Max Gerson, Big Medi$in subjected society to an exceedingly regrettable waste.

Dr. Gerson did not confine his practice to cancer, as he knew that all systemic "diseases" had a common cause.

I could easily fill several pages on Dr. Gerson, but that would lead us too far afield from our primary mission. If you are interested in gaining more insight into the Big C, as well as into a truly marvelous human being, read his book "A Cancer Therapy."

Max Gerson said that cancer occurs when the body has failed to produce an allergic inflammation. An "allergic inflammation," like other allergies, is a remedial event, the body's corrective action. Failure to produce that remedy is the result of failure of the liver and the other protective components of the physiology.

According to G. von Bergmann, M.D., a very eminent German physician, "...a cancer metabolism starts when the body is no longer able to produce a healing inflammation."

I will concede that cancer is a special condition. It is the ultimate failure of the body. What sets it apart from all other symptoms is that its last line of defense has been destroyed; hence its higher rate of fatality, its often-hopeless status.

Cancer is not a spontaneous happening; far from it. Research scientists estimate that it begins to develop some 15 years before its clinical diagnosis. So you can see why cancer is such a tough adversary, and also why, if we wish to be healthy and enjoy a long and vigorous life, we must not only accept, but rather relish, the responsibility of living right beginning at an early age and not depend on somebody to some day cut, poison, and burn a tumor out of our body.

At this point let us elaborate on Dr. Gerson's explanation of cancer. Your inner works, especially your liver, have the responsibility of maintaining your health. They constantly monitor your physiology and do whatever is necessary to keep you perking along. This is how we produce healing inflammations to restore homeostasis. When the inflammation, or symptom, has completed its job and is no longer needed, it fades away and we're feeling okay again. But unfortunately, if the body is abused too flagrantly and too long, all its components are affected, and those include the liver, the gall bladder, the kidneys, and all the rest. What was once a super-efficient filter is now clogged up from having to filter out too much junk for too long without the opportunity to maintain its own working condition. Now, when these guardian angels are finally disabled after years of abuse, who's going to do their job? Nobody. Sorry; it's too late. The poor patient has exhausted his last hope and his prospects for recovery look pretty grim. If he is to survive, something extraordinary must be done.

But there is some hope. Mother is so faithful to you and so intelligent and capable that if you're still half-alive with cancer, and given proper help, she can often turn your health around almost immediately. You may not see the improvement immediately, because a certain deficit must be made up before you arrive at the positive side of health, much as you won't see an overflow until the cup is full. But this is not a do-it-yourself project. Being a special condition, cancer requires special treatment by special experts.

I realize that many readers will look askance at me for the views I'm about to express, but these views are not arbitrary; they forced their way into my psyche over long eventful years. I do not, indeed cannot, look favorably on the conventional treatments for cancer. I have watched and studied their methods and results. I saw five of my friends killed by chemotherapy in two months. One celebrity has his cancer arrested by the cut, poison, and burn methods, and the whole world hears about it. But we don't hear about the numerous failures of those torturous and demoralizing methods. No, thank you!

This is not to say that I summarily vouch for the several nature-oriented cancer clinics in Mexico. But I do say I favor the concepts of their treatments, because they try to help Mother rather than fight against her in her attempts to heal. They recognize that cancer is a whole-body disease.

I've had the dubious privilege of spending a week at Genesis West, a cancer clinic in Mexico just south of the California border, not as a cancer patient but mostly to observe how these clinics operate. I hope Genesis West is not representative of the other clinics in Mexico. All of its ex-patients seem to be as disillusioned and regretful as I am about having gone there. Its owner, Jacob Swilling, Ph.D., originally of South Africa, delivers a fine lecture on cancer and expresses an admirable philosophy on it, but in his practice his patients and ex-patients seem unanimous in feeling deceived and shortchanged. I regret having to issue an unfavorable report on Genesis West, but would regret even more knowing that a reader of mine went there without the warning I owed him.

While I do not feel qualified to pass judgment on any clinic or hospital I have not visited, I am impressed by the reputation of the Contreras Clinic in Mejico. Contreras is reputed to be a capable and conscientious physician of fine character.

It should be no surprise to you when I say my number-one choice for the treatment of cancer is the Gerson Institute; Box 430; Bonita, CA 91908; (619) 472-7450. It is operated by Charlotte Gerson, daughter of the late Dr. Max Gerson. I have known of the Gerson people for some 40 years and have come to respect them profoundly, not only for their work on cancer, but for any chronic disease, because of their "body-totality" approach to treatment. The Gerson Institute does not own or operate any hospital but does work closely through the Mexican hospital in Baja California.

These American-operated cancer clinics are not only in Mexico but also in the Caribbean islands. They have sought refuge in foreign lands because our politicians, official and unofficial, representing Big Medi$in, will not allow them to save lives in the U.S. Oh, they'll give all kinds of reasons why these clinics are barred from the U.S., but the true reasons are so obvious that nothing can be resolved by discussing the matter any further.

In fairness to the alternative clinics, whatever may be their reputation, we must remember that an overwhelming majority of the cases who seek their help are already "terminal" when the patient first arrives there.

This is too critical a controversy for one person to decide for another. But I can say that you'll probably never have to choose between them if you resolve to live by Mother's laws.

In summary, cancer develops as do the other symptoms, except that the adverse conditions of the body are allowed to continue until even the protective agents themselves are rendered helpless. Individuals vary in their propensity to produce healing inflammations. Some appear healthy and never "get sick" but surprise themselves and others by getting cancer "out of the blue."

You have probably noticed that this treatise on cancer has been mostly "political." Relatively little has been said of specific physiological factors because the factors are the same for all symptoms. After all, they're all part of the same one disease. But let me discuss one dietary factor often accused, usually correctly, as a major cause of cancer: dietary fat. It is well circulated knowledge that it increases the tendency toward cancer; and that is true given the manner in which most of us live. We entertain so many free radicals in our systems that the fats we take in are quickly oxidized and turn rancid, and we know that rancidity is an extremely potent carcinogen. But if we keep our bodies clean inside and out, we can consume a moderate and adequate amount of fat without flirting with the Big C.

And how do we keep ourselves clean? By minimizing free radicals and optimizing antioxidants. Observe a few other disciplines and we're in good shape. We'll come back to these later.

Here is something I would very much like you to do for yourself — and me. As I have suggested above, make a real effort to find and read "A Cancer Therapy," by Max Gerson, M.D. Then read "The American Experience of Dr. Max Gerson, Censured for Curing Cancer," by S.J. Haught, who at first had set out to expose a "quack." This second book is available from The Gerson Institute at the address given a few lines above. The price is $6.95 but the book was sent to me gratis when I wrote the Institute for information. I promise you, you will find these books a major reading experience. They will shed light not only on cancer and the medical industry, but perhaps more importantly also on man's inhumanity to man.

ARTHRITIS

I think I'll confide in you. I'm getting a bit self-conscious about saying the same old thing over and over every time we undertake a new symptom. But since it's one of my major theses, I'm going to say it again: There is only one disease, a degenerated body, and all those so-called "diseases" are but localized manifestations of the disease. Arthritis is no exception. The way we should handle it is no different from how we handle other symptoms: Get healthy. Arthritis is far simpler than Big Medi$in makes it out to be. Oh, there are ramifications of course, in fact more than I have the patience to listen to. All by itself it is an extremely complicated and sophisticated science. But, as with all the other "diseases," what for? A tempest in a teapot. What for? It makes some people sicker and some people richer.

I've decided to go into a brief discussion of arthritis mainly for the benefit of anyone who is not yet familiar with my philosophy of health and disease. If this is old hat to you, feel free to skip however much of the discussion you wish.

Please don't misunderstand. Perhaps I've exaggerated some. The high-tech science of arthritis is not completely without merit. It does offer some benefit to patients whose source of medical "help" has been limited to Big Medi$in.

And then that help is superficial and temporary relief with no deep-down benefit, in fact only a deepening of the basic misery. Thus the reward that Big Medi$in grants its faithful patrons, you might say, ranks as a distant consolation prize. But to those patients who trust their doctors more than they do Mother, what more can I say but "Good luck!"?

By and large, doctors whose lifestyle is determined by their powerful business agents either admit they don't know much about arthritis or they say arthritis has no cause and cannot be cured. And they are right when they talk about themselves; they don't know much, or at least they say they don't know much. They never cure anybody anyway. But practitioners of nature-oriented disciplines, especially in foreign lands, help Mother cure arthritis by the thousands of cases.

Describing and otherwise discussing symptoms in too much detail distracts from, and are inimical to, the primary purpose of this book. Besides, they are moot and merely complicate our purpose, like spinning your car wheels in a muddy rut. We just need to know how to be healthy and avoid chasing shadows.

Arthritis, like cancer and most other symptoms, affects the entire system long before it manifests itself. The extraneous deposits in the joints, which are nonmetabolic materials, are composed of substances unusable by the body. The organs and glands also are congested, because of deficient elimination of wastes, and in turn lose their efficiency in eliminating wastes from the body. Its easy to understand what can happen when garbage accumulates in any system. The successful treatment entails restoring healthy conditions to the entire body and then allowing the body's own life force to take care of the situation. And the treatment we're alluding to here is not cortisone or any

151

other chemical poison. The treatment is metabolic and in harmony with Mother's principles. Too simple an explanation? Then why doesn't Big Medi$in come up with a better one? For the same old reason they say or don't say many other things. Like, why did a dozen doctors decline to tell me I had a horrible case of hypoglycemia when I was half-dead, or at least half-way to the nut house? Do we have to go into stuff like that again?

Deposits in arthritic joints, for our purposes, are not unlike the plaque deposits in hardened arteries. The general cause is the same: free radicals in junk food and to a lesser extent, environmental toxins and inadequate nutrition. Without proper nourishment the synovial membrane is unable to carry on its normal task of exchanging trash for food, and so the trash is trapped and with chemical changes remains in the joints as arthritic deposits. But we don't need to know even these specific whys and wherefores. We need only to know how to prevent and get rid of arthritis, and that is the same general remedy for all symptoms: Live in harmony with Mother's laws. The body has the infallible ability to heal itself in response to cleanliness and nourishment, notwithstanding what Big Medi$in tells you. I know from experience.

I've told you that I had arthritis when I was young. I had it pretty bad too. Now, more than 40 years later, I have none of it at all. I couldn't care less why I had it or how Mother took care of it. I have other interesting things to occupy my time while I'm still in this fascinating world. After all, I've got only about 50 more years.

There is a cause of and there is a cure for arthritis. Thousands of "hopeless" patients roll into European clinics in wheelchairs and walk out a few weeks later leaving their wheelchairs at the clinics on piles of other obsolete wheelchairs and crutches. Does this mean that if you're sick and tired of your arthritis you should go to Europe for relief? Not at all. If you can find a good nature-loving practitioner, good. But if that's too difficult or inconvenient, you can do a pretty good job of it all by yourself. Take a genuine interest in the ways of health, read and adopt the health measures you'll find in the latter part of this book, and you should be on your way toward not only healthy joints but also a whole healthy body.

Once again, if you have arthritis and don't want to keep it, you merely need to get healthy.

CHOLESTEROL and ATHEROSCLEROSIS

Okay, let's talk about this one. It comes in for its share of misconceptions too. First, I stand here bold-faced and tell you that dietary cholesterol is not a major factor in serum cholesterol ratings. And serum cholesterol ratings are not a major factor in heart disease either. I also say that blocked arteries can be cleared without medicines (or surgery), if one is willing to discipline himself enough to get the job done. We'll discuss how later. If the regimen is too difficult, one may resort to chelation, a procedure which cleans out not only the coronary arteries but all blood vessels, including those that feed the brain. So you can see that senility, as well as other vascular ills, can be postponed or avoided entirely while one vigorously lives his 120 years. We'll have more on this later too.

Now, this is going to take a lot of explaining. So let's explain it.

First, it must be admonished that dietary fat is an essential part of proper nourishment and is produced by the body as required. And it is required for almost all physiological activities. When it is inadequate, the quality of all cells suffer.

153

Skin wrinkles. Eyes blur. Bones ache. Shoulders stoop. The whole body and mind age before their time. Cutting down moderately on fats is one thing but quite another to minimize their consumption close to zero.

Let me tell you two very true stories in which I was involved, or at least an observer. Both principals were my friends and also related to me by marriage.

The first one let's call Ollie. He was a highly capable and successful builder-contractor, a few years either side of forty, a rising star on the Hawaii construction scene. His products were impressively massive structures. Ollie had a severe case of atherosclerosis. Wealthy as he was, he did not go to the hospital, instead retaining the services of three doctors in rotating eight-hour shifts in his own luxurious home. I had not known Ollie very well, but because I liked him — everyone liked Ollie — I occasionally went to visit him at his bedside. He was very easy to know and we had some enjoyable conversations. On one of those visits my mother was with me, and when the doctor answered the doorbell and we asked how Ollie was doing, the doctor shook his head and said, "Terribly. All three of us doctors are thoroughly puzzled. We've never encountered anything like this. We've had Ollie on a completely fat-free diet for several weeks but his cholesterol is running away from us and still climbing." I don't recall what figures he gave us but they were, as I recall, astronomical. Ollie succumbed shortly after.

As my mother and I left Ollie's home after listening to the doctor's discouraging story, we both scratched our heads in puzzlement. It was the late fifties, and not very much was known about cholesterol. Nevertheless, we had to accept our new learning that the body makes its own cholesterol. In this case we tentatively concluded that Ollie's body, not being accustomed to such deprivation of dietary cholesterol, worked overtime in its effort to compensate for the shortage. We left that tentative conclusion on the back burner, as at that time we could do nothing else with it.

Then in 1974 I spent two weeks in Los Angeles as a house guest of a young man I'll call Stu. He was 21, five-six and a hard 145 pounds. Though he was Caucasian he seemed to be Chinese-oriented (Pun intended.), eventually marrying a Chinese girl from Singapore. He instructed in Kung Fu and except for drinking milk was a very strict vegetarian. His low-fat milk, according to him, came from a Chinese dairy operated by Mr. Lo Fat. Anyway, Stu was admirably obsessed with keeping his intake of dietary fat as low as possible. This, I told him, was not the way to go. But low-fat was in and Stu's diet was governed accordingly. Before leaving at the end of my visit I said, "Stu, one of these days you're going to have a medical exam, and when you do, you're going to be surprised with a very high serum cholesterol reading."

"No way. Where's the cholesterol coming from? You see for yourself I don't eat any fat."

"That's just it, Stu. Your body is going to overcompensate for what you should be giving it."

"Never happen, Bert. Never happen."

Well, in about a year Stu did have a medical exam and came away with a serum cholesterol reading of 395 mg/dl, as I recall. He was 22, and I at 54 had a reading of 195. And I had been eating, and still eat, a moderate amount of fat any time I took a fancy to, which was, and is, fairly often.

Now let's look at the other side of this coin. Dr. Fred Kern of the University of Colorado School of Medicine reports that an 88-year-old man has been eating between 20 and 30 eggs a day for the last 15 years and his cholesterol readings remain between 150 and 200 mg/dl, a very normal reading, in fact enviably low for a man his age. His LDL cholesterol is 142 and his HDL is 45. While this man's high consumption of eggs is a bit unusual, his cholesterol non-response to his diet is not surprising. I have known of more than a few such non-responses. For example, 100 men were put on a diet of 18 eggs per week for six months and ended with a lower average cholesterol reading than at the beginning of the study.

While egg yolks are high in cholesterol, reportedly they also contain eight times the amount of lecithin required to metabolize the cholesterol contained. In fact, eggs are supposed to be the richest known natural source of lecithin.

A chart published by the U.S. Department of Agriculture shows the increase in the incidence of heart attacks. Superimposed on the same chart is a graph showing the steep decline in egg consumption in recent years in response to the Great American Egg Scare. These two graphs cross in the middle of the chart as the heart attack line goes up and the egg consumption line goes down. To those who have fallen for the Scare, the chart must be a paradox. But the relative directions of these two graphs, while not technically conclusive, certainly suggest that the Egg Scare is a farce. I personally feel that a great many Americans are missing out on a wholesome and economical source of nourishment.

Also noteworthy is that the inhabitants of Soviet Georgia traditionally eat abundant quantities of fatty meats and whole milk products. And more centenarians are found here than in any other area of the world.

Why do so many contradictions exist in matters of diet and health in America? Given a fair degree of adherence to the so-called scientific method, and if all reports made are sincere, wouldn't you surmise that the extent of the contradictions would be far less? Well, in view of all the other axe-grinding contradictions, what should one expect? Moreover, it seems these days that scientific truths are not as important as politico-economic advantages. Take the tobacco industry for example. Almost everybody in America knows that tobacco is extremely harmful, while almost every executive officer in the industry tries to tell us that tobacco really isn't as bad as we think it is. Reports are bandied about as political footballs and altered at will, even in midflight, to deceive the opposition and the spectators as well. Winning is everything, and the truth be damned.

"Our best medical minds have told us for decades that dietary fat is responsible for blockage of coronary arteries, and you tell me they're wrong? I think this time you've gone too far, contradicting just to contradict. It seems everybody's out of step but you. If fat is not the villain, what is?"

Good question. I'm glad you asked. A while back we discussed free radicals and how their reactive nature causes all kinds of mischief throughout our systems. Well, here they are again, and making trouble again. They attack the cells of the artery linings and make them a good foundation for a calcified plaque which in turn is a good foundation for the build-up of cholesterol which together with the other components of the deposit are what cause hardening of the arteries, or arteriosclerosis. If conditions are optimal for cholesterol to adhere to the linings of the arteries, cholesterol will adhere no matter the concentration of the stuff in the blood. It doesn't take much cholesterol to block up the arteries; so there's no shortage of it, whether its serum reading is 120 or 360 mg/dl. And what largely determines the condition of the artery linings is the action of free radicals.

Free radicals further facilitate arterial blockage by rendering dietary fat rancid, and rancidity, besides being extremely carcinogenic, in turn renders fat more amenable to ending up on the linings of the arteries.

So the development of blockage of the coronary arteries, and other arteries as well, is not so much a matter of cholesterol as it is of free radicals — how much garbage one has circulating in his body. In still other words, conversely, the cleaner one's insides, other conditions being equal, the cleaner will his arteries tend to be.

In summary, filthy inners are more responsible for artery blockage than are dietary and blood serum cholesterol. And again, fat is an essential part of a good diet and its consumption should not be too drastically curtailed. If we keep our bodies clean inside and out, we can benefit from a moderate and adequate amount of fat without unduly fearing arteriosclerosis.

PROSTATITIS

Prostatitis, known also as BPH, benign prostatic hypertrophy, or benign prostatic hyperplasia, though a rampant men's malady, concerns, or should concern, millions of women as well. For in a close loving relationship what concerns one concerns the other, and in America prostatitis concerns an overwhelming majority of men middle-aged and older. Increasingly younger men are falling victims to their prostates too, undoubtedly because of our worsening lifestyle. The symptoms are frequent and difficult urination and sexual impotence. While statistically there seems to be no correlation between prostatitis and cancer of the prostate, it's only logical to assume that an enlarged and inflamed prostate gland will more readily yield to a malignancy than will a healthy one. It's also logical to assume that a sick gland is hosted by a sicker body than one that hosts a healthy gland. So prostatitis warrants all the attention and exposure we're willing to give it.

Let's forego the statistics on this humbug troublemaker. We'll use our space to talk about you and how you can keep your prostate healthy or if you are already a victim, how you can enhance its health. Neither do we need to go into all its ramifications, for so many men are familiar with them that to explain would probably be redundant.

Prostatitis is an extremely difficult condition to overcome. Most men can only hope to alleviate their discomfort, if they can even do that. Consequently, and understandably, many and probably most orthodox doctors will without hesitation recommend surgical removal of the gland at the first sign of enlargement. But please think hard and long before yielding to his scalpel, for prostatectomy is not by any means a romp in the park or exempt from risk and sacrifice. Don't let anybody add your precious prostate to the list of organs the doctors describe as a bunch of useless organs which Mother gave birth to by mistake, like your gallbladder, appendix, tonsils, and adenoids.

I've told you how sick I was in my youth. When I was about 32 my urologist detected an enlargement of my gland and matter-of-factly began to plan for my surgery, explaining that that was standard procedure. I told him he could have my prostate if he would let me take his. Today, thanks no doubt to better living habits, I still have my prostate and was told recently by my urologist that it was in fair shape, better than "normal" for my age.

Regretfully but realistically, I must render my opinion that if your prostate is slightly enlarged and you can keep it from further enlargement for the rest of your life, you'd be doing pretty well. If you can do better than that, bully-

bully for you! You must have exercised considerable character and discipline to do what you did.

Prostatitis is so stubborn that it is my firm opinion that nobody will ever overcome an existing case of it while remaining on the standard American diet, known also as SAD. If one is to succeed, he must adhere pretty closely to Mother's laws and live in harmony with natural conditions, and even then overcoming prostatitis would be a heroic feat.

Let's get down to what you can do for yourself to keep your prostate from giving you trouble as the years go by. First, of course, is to keep your whole body as healthy as possible. This is the only way I know of that will give you real, deep-down, benefit. Health measures will be discussed toward the end of this book. But there's nothing wrong with trying to get temporary relief and comfort, and that is done mostly with heat and exercise. You are probably familiar with the well-known sitz bath, in which one merely sits in a tub of hot water. The heat "loosens up" the gland and the surrounding tissues, ridding them of stagnation and encouraging circulation of blood and lymph; in other words, "bringing them alive." Exercise also enhances circulation and combats stagnation, which is a very essential part of and a prerequisite for prostatitis. Any measure that stimulates and enlivens the prostate and the surrounding tissues can benefit the situation. Many exercises have been suggested as therapy for the prostate, but your own imagination in innovating your own exercises which have greater meaning to you could be more beneficial. Nevertheless I will explain here a few "classic" exercises for your consideration:

Alternately tighten and relax the sphincter muscles several times in a series and do several series every day.

The muscles we're talking about are the ones we use to stop the flow of urine. After warming up to this exercise a few days, do it as often and as vigorously as your common sense dictates. I enthusiastically suggest that you do it every time you pee and that you sit down to pee. Sitting down to pee is a great thing to do even if you have a healthy prostate, but especially convenient and comfortable for the victim of prostatitis. I grant you it will be difficult to maintain your enthusiasm for the project, especially if you have to carry it alone, but try to remember what we learned in grade school, that perseverance conquers all.

Lying on your back, grasp both feet by their outside edges and pull them toward your crotch area. (You can enhance your grip by wrapping your little toes between your thumbs and index fingers.) This will force your knees outward and you should feel a strong tension in the general area of your crotch. This action is intended to wake up your prostate from its hibernation. Pull and relax several times, striving for strong tension in your crotch area, where you know your prostate is. Feel free to alter the exercise any which way you can to produce a better pull. For example, you might straighten your legs while still holding on to your feet and do a split. While in this variation you might alternately bend your knees and straighten them. Do anything that will give you not only a strong pull but also a varying direction of pull and perhaps in a slightly differing location.

Then there's the duck waddle. Walk around in a deep squat on flat feet. Again, use your good judgment.

Some practitioners advise their patients to make a habit of pounding their own buttocks with the thumb side of their fists. Anything to enliven the general area.

161

If you're not familiar with foot reflexology, do get familiar with it. Get yourself a good reflex chart and go to work on the reflex areas for your prostate. If you question the validity of the art, I personally vouch for it. Is it worth the hassle of trying something new? I guess it depends on how much you value your prostate.

Let me tell you what food supplementation is recommended for your prostate by Dr. Jonathan V. Wright in his valuable book "Dr. Wright's Book of Nutritional Therapy":

1. Chelated zinc: 50 mg, 1 tablet 3 times daily.

2. Essential fatty acids capsules: 400 mg, 1 capsule 3 times daily.

3. Tablets made from whole animal prostate gland: 2 tablets 3 times daily.

4. Bee pollen: 3 tablets daily.

Zinc and essential fatty acids are contained in seeds and nuts. Raw pumpkin seeds and raw sunflower seeds are especially rich in them. Eat a handful of either or each every day.

Two other highly recommended supplements are pygeum africanum, extracted from an African pine tree; and saw palmetto, extracted from the saw palmetto plant which grows profusely along the southeastern coast of North America. In a negative vein, I should tell you this: Almost every histaminic drug sold for the relief of allergies will aggravate a diseased prostate gland. If you take one of these, you will probably experience an acute swelling of your gland. Read the printing on the package and you will find the precaution, but it will be inconspicuously buried in the fine print.

Numerous health food providers market organic supplements compounded especially for the prostate. They all are approximately similar and their analyses look good. But whether you should buy these supplements or how much you should buy I guess depends on the degree of the enlargement of your prostate, how intent you are on improving your condition, and your financial condition. However you handle your project, it'll be a slow go. As I have said, all you can realistically hope for is to keep your gland from enlarging further, or perhaps achieve moderate improvement of the condition. If you hope to obtain a real cure, you're going to have to let Mother do it and you'll have to give her your full cooperation.

If I haven't given you the encouragement you had hoped for, it's because I realize the stubborn nature of prostatitis and would not want to be guilty of exaggerating the prospects of a cure. But I say again, keep your prostate in check and you'll have a victory of sorts. If you're very conscientious, responsible, and willing to pay the price, there is nothing to say you can't do much better.

HYPOGLYCEMIA and DIABETES

Hypoglycemia, known also as low blood sugar, is the one that wrecked my life, as well as the lives of millions of others. As syphilis used to be, it is a great imitator. Moreover, it is a wellspring of numerous other maladies, meaning that without an underlying condition of hypoglycemia certain other symptoms could not develop. This is because hypoglycemia, whose essential condition is a short supply of sugar in the blood, maintains a condition of the body that is conducive to the development of various other imbalances. A few of these symptoms (Notice that I said symptoms, not diseases.) are hay fever, asthma, frequent colds, depression, alcoholism, rheumatic fever, ulcers, neuroses, fatigue, anxiety, schizophrenia, addictions of all kinds. I have just spouted out a mouthful. How is it that a layman like me knows all this stuff while doctors don't? Many doctors do know it, but because hypoglycemia is a stepchild of Big Medi$in, most doctors don't want to know it. If you're even moderately well versed on hypoglycemia, you probably know that most doctors try to tell patients that it is nothing but a fad or a figment of the imagination. They also say that hypoglycemics are hypochondriacs. If these statements are not true, why in the world do doctors make them? You probably know.

I have averred that hypoglycemia is a stepchild of Big Medi$in. It's an unwanted stepchild because when it is correctly diagnosed and treated, health results. And, as you well know, health is the big enemy of Big Medi$in. Compounding the disadvantage to the doctor, even the treatment of this malady is profitless to him, because the only sensible remedy is an improvement in the diet of the patient, and the doctor doesn't deal in groceries. Even if he could, he wouldn't, because the profit in food is downright piddling alongside the fat fees charged for medical services. And when health develops, there goes another series of fat fees. How do I know all these wild and not-so-funny facts? These wild and not-so-funny facts happened to me.

Hypoglycemia is not a black-or-white condition. It is experienced in varying degrees. On this basis, many authorities estimate that more than half of Americans have it. This is hardly surprising in view of the piles of junk we (not including me, please) stuff into our faces. I hope you're not included either.

This is a good time to introduce my philosophy on "being good to myself and partaking of the enjoyable things of life." If one is not willing to sacrifice for his health, if he is not willing to pay the price, I guess he must expect some degree of poor health. But of course it's his choice. Here is the rationalization which helps me succeed to a moderate degree in maintaining a tolerable lifestyle: (Of course I have the advantage of having been through the crucible of extreme hypoglycemia and had the good fortune of being able to see what two and two add up to.) Whatever superficial and temporary jollies I sacrifice for my health are more than made up for by the self respect I gain by my discipline. And when God gives me a big hug and pats me on the back, that does it.

Look again at those symptoms I listed above as offsprings of hypoglycemia. Notice that they all are very chronic illnesses. Their victims keep going to the doctor forever and never really get their problems resolved, and that is because their integrating factor, hypoglycemia, has not been resolved and is still hanging on to them. Let's see now: All those symptoms, times several million patients, times a thousand bucks per patient; we're beginning to talk big money. Listen. Why would anyone want to diagnose hypoglycemia? I guess I was wrong when I said hypoglycemia was Big Medi$in's stepchild. It must be one of its favorite children, as long as it is not acknowledged.

It does seem, doesn't it, that I'm derogating Big Medi$in? I'm really not. I'm merely stating the facts as I know them to be, after years of experience and observation. It is the facts themselves that reflect on the entities involved. I reluctantly present them here because you and many millions of others need the truth and insight if you are to exercise your rights as members of my human family. I want you to leave the darkness and come walk in the sunlight.

How does hypoglycemia happen? When the healthy pancreas senses the presence of sugar in the blood, it releases the hormone insulin to metabolize the sugar and convert it into energy for use or storage. And it does so in amounts proportional to the amount of sugar present. But not everybody has a healthy pancreas. Some pancreases are hypersensitive, and that condition is hypoglycemia, in which excessive amounts of insulin are released by the pancreas.

In general, one becomes hypoglycemic by abusing his pancreas, and he does that by overloading it with sugar, not necessarily the beautiful white stuff but sugar in all forms. Don't be so sure I'm not talking about you, because the average American consumes about five-eighths of a cup of sugar per day, some from his beloved sugar bowl but mostly hidden, and not so hidden, in processed foods.

Specialists have categorized hypoglycemia into two types: organic and functional. The organic type is a result of actual physical damage to the pancreas and is far less common than the functional. In the functional, the pancreas is not damaged and there seems to be no real consensus on its cause. But we do know that sugar is a common denominator, and regardless of the cause, sugar management is critical.

What happens in the body of a hypoglycemic? First, the excessive amounts of insulin metabolize the sugar so fast that the body finds itself short of sugar and energy and thus cannot function as it should. As in the physical world nothing happens without energy, so in the hypoglycemic many intended functions are left unfulfilled. The body cries for energy, the brain gets the message, and thus an addict is born or maintained in his addiction. The brain, which relies solely on blood sugar, more specifically termed glucose, for its energy, is curtailed in its ability to function, much as an engine stops when it runs out of fuel. Imbalances in the body chemistry give rise to an almost infinite number of physiological malfunctions; hence the long string of symptoms listed above, plus many more not listed. As related in the chapter College of Hard Knocks, my entire scholastic career was utterly destroyed by hypoglycemia. When the brain is starved for food, believe me, it's miserable. Many good books have been written on the subject, but one of my favorites is "Body, Mind and Sugar," by Dr. E.M. Abrahamson and A.W. Pezet. It's an old one but still respected as a classic work today. In short, a healthy diet for a "normal" person is generally a healthy diet for a hypoglycemic. Remember the "oneness" of the body.

A special note to my fellow hypoglycemics: If you are duly adhering to the standard protocol for hypoglycemia; namely, that you eat about six smaller meals spaced closer together rather than the usual three big meals spaced about six hours apart, your dietary regimen must be more stringent than that of a "normal" person. Your system is busy digesting food close to twenty hours every day, and the early morning hours are the only time it is free of that task. Since a system in the process of digestion is too occupied to be able to give much attention to the task of rejuvenating the body, there's not much time for housecleaning and other metabolic operations. This situation no doubt contributes considerably to the many miseries of hypoglycemics. I hope you can see that you're at a disadvantage and must compensate for it. Because you don't have much time for throwing out trash, the smart thing to do is to have less trash to throw out, and to do that you must put less in.

Diabetes is on the opposite side of the hypoglycemic coin. It exists when the pancreas fails to produce and release insulin in sufficient quantities to adequately metabolize dietary sugar. The result, of course, is excessive concentrations of sugar in the blood and tissues of the entire body. Some of the sugar is excreted in the urine but not enough of it to normalize the problem. Though diabetes and hypoglycemia are direct opposites in cause and effect, understanding the nature of one increases understanding of the other, for the characteristics of these two maladies complement each other like hand and glove. It should be noted that if a hypoglycemic fails to alleviate his problem and also allows it to worsen, he becomes a candidate for diabetes. One factor shared by these two patients is excessive intake of sugar.

We've spoken a lot about junk food, of which sugar is one of the worst. The poor diabetic harbors a preponderance of big-time junk in his body even when he religiously tries to avoid it. And so he is subject to the many ills for which junk is responsible, including atheroscleroisis. This is why he is so vulnerable to gangrene and all other infections. There's no telling how many feet and legs have been lost to gangrene and how many lives have been ravaged and shortened by diabetes.

As one who recognizes the power of the body to at least mitigate the ills which befall it, I can generalize what I would do as a diabetic: First I would seek the services of a practitioner who is willing to work with Mother rather than against her. This is what he would probably do for me or advise me to do for myself: Keep myself as clean as possible inside and out, and this entails occasional colonic irrigations when deemed advisable; avoid junk foods, especially sugar and other refined carbohydrates; maintain in my body a goodly supply of antioxidants to minimize the effects of the free radicals which so adversely affect diabetics; try my very best to observe all of Mother's rules for health.

This is not to say you should not also seek the help of a conventional MD if you feel you need him. After all, you may have a real need for insulin supplementation. But your efforts to keep healthy will make the MDs treatment more effective.

I can't resist the obvious fact that the best way to treat diabetes is to not let it get to you in the first place, and I don't have to tell you how to do that.

OBESITY

In 1991, 30,000,000 American women were size 14 or larger. That's one-third of all adult American women.

While I do not pretend to be very knowledgeable on obesity, I can say a few things about it with confidence. I have had considerable experience with my body and have a fair idea of how it works.

I do not agree with people who say, "What determines whether you gain or lose weight is the difference between the amount of energy in the food you consume and the amount of energy you expend. It's that simple." It's not that simple. Such statements spring not only from a lack of understanding of physiology but also a lack of compassion for our chubby friends.

I will say this: Of all the theories put forth to account for obesity, I believe the most reliable is that when non-metabolic materials (junk) are deposited as sludge in the body, the glands and other organs, being part of the body, are included as sites of deposit. They lose varying degrees of their efficiency, depending on how badly they are congested. Since they are responsible for the smooth operation of the body, including the deposition and maintenance of the proper amounts of material as part of the body, the loss of efficiency results in various imbalances in the workings of the body, including loss of ability to accurately govern the amounts of flesh and fat in and on the body. Some people lose weight, some gain. In the long run, a clean smooth-running physiology properly nourished will tend to maintain the ideal weight for a person. Have you ever seen an obese or skinny healthy person?

You might well respond with, "People's metabolisms, even healthy ones, are not all alike. Yours may keep you skinny but mine may keep me fat." I disagree again. If healthy physiologies differ that much between some of the Slim Jims and Fatsos I have seen, one would think that a few of us would have only one ear while some others would have three or four. It's not the innate character of physiology that makes it malfunction. Rather it's its less-than-healthy condition that's responsible. Have you noticed that infants, before their systems are corrupted by the Standard American Diet (SAD), differ very little in body proportion?

You just can't keep smoking and stuffing your face with junk and expect to be trim as a race horse.

Now, if you are obese, I would like to reward you for your patience and courtesy in listening to a skinny fellow who has never walked in your shoes. I am going to entertain you with a little narrative which should be more than entertaining in that it holds the potential for a significant loss of weight.

Some time in the early sixties my friend Earl lent me an old book by the late once-famed Dr. Henry Lindlahr. It was written just after the turn of the century, 1905 or so, and dealt with what the author called the "catabolic diet." "Catabolic" refers to a negative energy balance. The diet is a sure-fire way to lose weight in that it requires more energy to digest than the energy it provides. Sound great? It is great. For a refreshing change you can now get something for nothing, or more accurately, lose something for nothing.

When I returned the book to Earl a few days later, he said to me, "I now weigh 170 pounds. In thirty days I will

be down to 140. You watch my catabolic diet in action."
At the end of the 30 days Earl had obviously lost some
weight. I asked, "Well, Earl, did you make it?" He smiled
sheepishly and said rather apologetically, "Naw, I lost only
20 pounds, but at least I'm down to 150. He was about five-
foot-four, still a bit chubby, but he had demonstrated what
can be done with a little effort and the catabolic diet.

If you would like to emulate Earl and shed some of your
own blubber, here's what you should do: Make your diet
predominantly fresh raw vegetables, mostly green. Minimize
the salad dressing. Eat as much as you wish. The more you
eat of these veggies, the more you will lose. Since the diet is
chock-full of vitamins and minerals, it is comparatively safe
if not carried on too long.

The raw vegetables will do three good things for you: (1)
nourish you, (2) make you lose weight, and (3) detoxify
you, including your organs, rendering them more efficient
in regulating your weight — and health. Good luck!

Let me state one more truism on the subject: If obese
people have shorter lives, it's not only the overweight, per
se, that kills them prematurely. The less-than-healthy
physiology that made them obese in the first place must
share part of the responsibility for the early demise.

Obese man to druggist: "You got any talcum powder?"
Druggist: "Sure do. Walk this way, please."
Obese man: "If I could walk that way, you think I
would need talcum powder?"

CONSTIPATION and DIARRHEA

Constipation is the inability of the body's mechanism,
by way of its alimentary system, to relieve itself of waste
matter often enough and in sufficient quantities to maintain

171

a healthy condition of itself. The following are among the major causes of the difficulty.

1. Insufficient dietary fiber. This is probably the most cited cause of constipation. And the simplest way to get enough fiber is to eat most of one's food in as natural a state as possible; in other words, food that has been minimally processed by man. That means mostly fruits and vegetables, mostly raw, and unprocessed whole cereal grains, mostly cooked.

2. Processed foods. Minimize their consumption, because they have been robbed of many of their beneficial components and because they have been adulterated with harmful chemicals. They give rise to free radicals, plenty of them. They also create an unnatural condition in the intestines, which in turn encourages the establishment of bacterial populations inimical to the normal and desired functions of the intestines. These undesirable microbes, especially the now-notorious Escherichia coli, monopolize the intestinal space and crowd out the beneficial bacteria, the most well-known of which is Lactobacillus acidophilus. E. coli is a cesspool bacterium; so you can imagine what goes on in the intestines when a faulty diet helps the bad guys take over the intestines and throw the entire body into turmoil. With the tone of the physiology thus undermined, peristalsis, the process which moves the food waste through the intestines and out of the body, loses its efficiency and sometimes shuts down altogether. The result of this condition is constipation.

3. Time restrictions. These restrictions are imposed on us by ourselves and by society, of which occupational employment is a major part. When Mother says, "Go to the bathroom," and we don't go, what can she do but shut

down the peristaltic action? You should be thankful she doesn't ignore your negligence and allow you to disgrace yourself. If you too often call for a shutdown, the peristalsis will tend to lose its efficiency and result in a backlog of compacted garbage, toxemia, and disease. This unhealthy state does very little for the cause of good health and increases the incidence of colorectal cancer and hemorrhoids.

I have said all along that I am just sharing my thoughts with you, not telling you how you should live your life. But now I will extend myself and say that if you don't relish the specter of carrying a portable toilet around with you under your garment, I strongly suggest that you take especial care of your eliminative machinery right now. As has been often and correctly said, "Death begins in the colon."

We have already discussed diarrhea but let's push it once more. It is one of Mother's means of cleaning out the body when it harbors more toxins than it can handle by normal means. I hope you respect and appreciate her enough to not try to frustrate her efforts by swallowing chemical "remedies." Should she be called on to do a cleaning job on you, help her along by drinking plenty of water and eating sparingly and only of "clean" foods.

It would behoove you to drink six to eight glasses of good, clean water every day. If your eliminative system and function are sub-par, here's some advice that should yield gratifying results: First thing in the morning, drink a full glass, or preferably two, of water. After a few minutes have some fruit as your first food of the day. Or, if you're conscientious and in real need of improvement, try an all-day water fast followed by an all-day fruit fast.

I can easily understand that social situations sometimes do occur that require the closing of the garbage chute by eliminating the production of wash water. In such cases when you have no choice, you should take measures to compensate for your adverse actions by making especial efforts to get back into general health. You know how to do that.

The healthy person defecates twice a day and dispenses about two pounds of the stuff. If you don't believe that, you will when you get healthy. Ever wonder what happens to all that junk people stuff into their faces when they "go" only once in two or three days? Is it any mystery why the American market is loaded with remedies such as deodorants, breath fresheners, dandruff stoppers, antiperspirants, athlete's foot sprays, not to mention practically every other medicine designed by man to remedy all manner of physical ills?

Let me tell you more about junk:

Some of it escapes through the pores, some in the breath, a lot turns to fat, and a lot gets in line behind all the previous junk that can't get out of the body because our bodies lack the capacity to purge such an abnormal accumulation of waste. When enough junk saturates the body, the organs, especially the liver, get their share of it and lose their efficiency. When they get sufficiently disabled, that's when someone says, "Didja hear about Elmer? He's got a malignancy."

Remember, the liver is the first and last defender of the body. When it's knocked out of the game, the only way to restore real health before too late is to restore it to health and you do that by restoring the whole body, and you do that not with a knife, synthetic chemicals, or zapping the body with destructive rays. You do that only by being a Prodigal Son and helping Mother.

ALCOHOLISM

"If you haven't walked in my shoes, get the hell off my back! You don't begin to know anything about me and my problem."

No, I haven't walked in your shoes, but I have walked close to persons who have walked in your shoes; so I have a pretty good idea of your difficulties. Moreover, I have a load of compassion for you. We are still brothers and sisters, and because of that, what hurts you hurts me, not only because of your miseries but also because your actions so very adversely impinges on the lives and fortunes of those close to you.

Alcoholism is essentially a cry for nourishment, down at the cellular level. The starvation behind the symptom is most commonly an integral part of hypoglycemia, or low blood sugar. Dr. E. M. Abrahamson and A. W. Pezet in their highly respected book "Body, Mind and Sugar" relate how they have never found an alcoholic who didn't also have hypoglycemia. They also tell of cases where alcoholics have shed their craving for alcohol with the administration of a wholesome diet.

Having experienced the credibility of their work, and also having encountered other impressive indications of the validity of the concept, I am thoroughly convinced that, as Abrahamson and Pezet have said, "...in alcoholism, as in the other allergies, hyperinsulinism (another term for hypoglycemia) is a necessary underlying condition."

As convincing as the evidence is of the validity of the concept that hypoglycemia is a necessary condition for alcoholism, and also because many researchers have set forth the concept for public perusal, I find it extremely puzzling that no establishment entities of significance have picked up the ball and tried to enlighten the alcoholic community

175

of the potential benefit of the concept. Alcoholics Anonymous still uses will power and tricks of the mind in trying to maintain sobriety. Despite their stalwart efforts, a pathetically small minority of them truly succeed.

It is significant also that, from what I can gather, alcoholics fighting the addiction, including those at the AA meetings, consume substantial quantities of coffee, sweet pastries, and tobacco. It is well known that hypoglycemics also use these crutches in their efforts to satiate their cravings for the energy which is normally provided by blood glucose in a healthy body. Unfortunately, this practice only exacerbates the problem, and the poor victim is trapped in a vicious circle.

I implore all alcoholics, as well as victims of other phantom maladies, to look into the possibility that hypoglycemia is indeed at the base of their problems, or at least consider that a healthy diet, free of excessive refined carbohydrates and providing adequate energy, may very well alleviate their need for surrogate and artificial nutrition.

In closing I must tell you about dear Peggy Boyd. She was once an alcoholic. (In your language, she still is.) After fighting the devil and herself for years, she found a "secret weapon," which was to first relieve herself of her hypoglycemia. And she did that by achieving good, robust health. But the ingredients for the kind of real, deep-down health needed to relieve the alcoholic are not run-of-the-mill everyday items. So I'll give you her toll-free telephone number and mailing address at her store which she got into because of the enthusiasm she experienced through her escape from alcohol. If you appreciate friendly, sympathetic, and helpful people, you will enjoy speaking with Peggy. You will find her a generous fountainhead of valuable information on health. Ask her about her "Secret

Weapon Pep-Up Drink." You can either order it from her or you can ask her for the recipe, which she generously gives out.

I have never personally met the lady and I have no axe to grind. Here's how to get hold of her:

Peggy's Health Store
1-800-862-9191
151 First Street
Los Altos, CA 94022
Good Luck!

STRESS

The Superior Tool Company has struggled for years with a problem which has cut deeply into its profits and in fact seriously threatens the marketability of its best-selling product, a machine that is still on the market only because of its exceptional usefulness and the protection afforded by its patent. Were a similar machine available from some other manufacturer, Superior Tool would have lost all its customers for this machine by now.

The machine, named Do-All, is a marvel of ingenious design and all-in-all has been a great boon to it's users, Superior's customers. The problem is that its users have been breaking a primary lever on the machine by pulling too hard on the handle and exerting excessive stresses on the lever. Superior, over the 15 years it has marketed Do-All, has had to replace at its own expense more than 60 percent of the levers of all the Do-Alls it has sold, some of them more than once. To alleviate the difficulty they have advised thousands of customers on the art of pulling on the handle, trying to convince them that it can be pulled with less gusto and without sacrificing too much of the machine's efficiency and production time. "You're not pulling correctly," is their routine advice.

One young employee who helps make this lever has made several suggestions to his superiors; such as improving the composition of the alloy that goes into the casting of the lever, forging the lever instead of casting it, making it from heavy steel plate instead of casting it, changing the ratios of the moment arms in the linkages so that less force on the lever would be required to operate the machine, and adding a reinforcing rib near the base of the lever. But his superiors, with degrees from renown engineering schools, consider the young man's suggested remedies too simple and low-tech. "Nothing wrong with the lever. Reduce the stresses and it'll be okay. The stresses are the problem, not the lever. If we could only get the customers to use the machine correctly..."

Superior's competitors are already planning to manufacture and market similar machines, because they realize the patent on it will not run forever.

If this stupid story reminds you of a similarly stupid situation in the realm of human health care, you and I are on the same frequency. Have you noticed that many people, even the educated ones in white frocks and plush offices, cast not an iota of suspicion toward the structure being stressed? They seem to regard the mind and emotions as an ethereal mystical aura floating a few inches above our heads. They know that the mind and emotions are a product of the brain but that seems to be as far as they will go. The body is too mundane to consider. It's more cultured and respectable to contemplate the profundities of the mystical mind.

The mind and emotions are literally, not figuratively, electrical impulses produced in the brain. We can stop the production by resting the brain, deciding to refrain from thinking. The brain is a major integral part of an electrical system we call our nerves, which are physical objects which can be seen, felt, cut, and pinched. They need to be nurtured like the rest of the body. There are healthy nervous systems and there are unhealthy ones.

Stresses are a normal and healthy part of living. Without them we don't grow. They are sometimes called growing pains. Some philosophical souls express this concept by saying, "The kite goes up against the wind." or "Adversity builds character." To eliminate stress is to withhold food from our minds, though, as in other aspects of life, we don't want stresses which our bodies and minds cannot tolerate. If we strengthen our bodies and minds, our normal, healthy stresses will remain normal and healthy and not become excessive. Not only that; our bodies and minds would be fortified against all other maladies which would otherwise rear their ugly heads. Make sense?

And what of the currently popular "chronic fatigue syndrome?" Same old story. Oh yes, the medical pundits tack sophisticated and erudite explanations to this humbug symptom, but the basic cause is always the same — an enervated, degenerated, and deteriorated physiology. Stress, fatigue, "nerves" — they're all the same, just additional holes in the same old rotten, leaky bag. Ho hum...

So you can see that a healthy, strong body with its healthy, strong nervous system, including the brain, will be better able to handle stress.

179

Chapter Five

Caveat Emptor

The old man had always been pretty quiet, in fact almost out of contact with the rest of the town. The young people knew him as just Bill, the old geezer who was always on the old bench in front of the old store, just part of the scenery. Bill seemed to be about 85; no one really knew. He had been widowed about 20 years now, having lost his wife to cancer. Obviously he was now just waiting on destiny.

About a dozen young men were "hanging out" in front of the store, not having much to say about anything, except now and then what a dead, good-for-nothing town they lived in. "How in the hell did it ever get the name 'Pleasant'"? mocked one of them, not really asking.

This was when old Bill spoke up, surprising everyone within earshot. His larynx had been out of use for so long that his voice was weak. But what he lacked in volume he easily made up for by his facial and tonal expressions. "Listen, you young citizens of this great little town..."

"Great little town!" Several of the youths responded in unison.

"As I was beginning to say, Listen! Pleasant wasn't always this pitiful. This used to be a very fine town. I know, because I helped build it — from scratch. You there, young Jensen, listen. Your grandfather and I were like brothers, and I loved him like one. We and a few others like us wanted a good, wholesome place to live in and bring up our children.

So we built Pleasant, carefully, one family at a time. This town didn't just happen. No, sir. We built it the way we wanted it. And it deserved its name."

The young men were now filled with quiet excitement — and new respect for the old man. Some of them had never heard Bill utter a word, let alone bring up the ancient past.

"Was it better than it is now?" one asked. Bill didn't feel the need to answer. He just kept looking to one side and nodding his head. Obviously in deep reminiscence. The same boy asked, "Well, what happened, Bill?"

"Greed! That's what happened." It was almost a yell, the loudest Bill had sounded off probably for years, maybe decades. "Greed and lack of love. That's all it was. You see, after a few dozen families had moved out of Capitalia into Pleasant, some businessmen in Capitalia began to see certain opportunities in our growing little town. More and more they came over trying to sell us this and that. Most of their ideas were not what we wanted for our town, and we told them so. But they kept trying. For example, when they wanted to build that big fancy country club they now have in Capitalia, where they wanted it was where their garbage dump used to be. So they came over to Pleasant and tried to get us to accept their garbage. 'Nosiree,' we told them. 'We have garbage of our own. We don't need yours!' Well, those hustlers never gave up. They got some professional experts and psychologists from New York and kept working on us. Well, they finally sorta succeeded. They convinced us that their garbage would some day be valuable, usable land if we would let them dump the stuff in the gully between those two ridges on the high side of town. You know, where all the junk piles are and nobody goes there anymore? Well, you may not know this but that junk is full of dangerous poisons. You know why we have that beautiful expensive water treatment plant in town now? Because that trash from Capitalia poisoned our water. But that wasn't enough. They even talked us into paying them for giving us their poisons. That's how clever some people can be when they're chasing the buck. But don't ask me how they pulled it off. I was dead set against it, even when they brought their high-class chemists to show us that their poisons were really nothing. But some people here seemed to think the dump was good business for Pleasant. Some of you young fellas, go talk to your parents and grandparents about it. They may know.

"But that old dump isn't the whole story. Businessmen from Capitalia and other towns kept coming to Pleasant with their axes to grind, and it wasn't long before Pleasant was like any other town. All through the years a few of us tried very hard to protect our people from what they called progress. We were called all kinds of names; like old-fashioned, prudes, health nuts, and what-not. Well, eventually we all realized we couldn't fight greed and deceit anymore and finally gave up. I'm sure old Bob Jensen died of a broken heart. Many of us old-timers are still broken-hearted over the corruption of what was once a lovely, wholesome town.

"So you ask, 'What happened?' And I'm telling you greed happened. Greed from Capitalia, greed from other towns, and greed right here in Pleasant. Not only greed, but also deceit and gullibility, lack of common sense. Too much faith in all those people who were really only after our money and feeding us all kinds of wrong information.

"So why am I telling you all this? Because some of you up-and-coming young fellas will be leaders in Pleasant one of these days soon, and this is my last chance to try and save our beloved Pleasant. Perhaps you will be able to return it somewhere close to where it used to be. I've watched you boys grow up and I know some of you care about having a healthy town for yourselves, your future families, and everybody else in Pleasant. And I'm telling you that Pleasant isn't dead yet, only sick. I'm also telling you that you won't be able to restore wholesome conditions by bringing in outside help. You must build from the inside. Restore solid values within our people. Build hope and morale. Educate our children well, not only with books in school, but in the ways of life. If you care enough you can do all this.

"Okay, young men of Peasant. My time's over. I've tried my best but failed. The job is yours, and I'm expecting you to do better than I did. And always remember that you don't have to accept what others try to give you. Think for yourselves and skipper your own ship. As Bob Jensen and I used to say, Caveat emptor! Good night and good luck."

CHAPTER SIX

PROFITABLE IGNORANCE

One neighbor had a beautiful thick green weed-free lawn while the one next-door had a scrawny one with weeds all over the place. Mr. Greenlawn knew that Mr. Weedpatch spent a lot of time, energy, and money on his patch but was doing everything wrong. He didn't want to give his neighbor unsolicited advice, because Weedy was a college graduate and seemed to know everything. One day in desperation Weedy asked Greeny, "How in the world do you keep your lawn so healthy and beautiful? And with not much work at that?" That was enough to give Greeny reason to be a good neighbor and share his knowledge and expertise.

"Glad you asked, Weedy. I guess you might say I eliminate the negative and accentuate the positive. Meaning I just keep my grass healthy by feeding it well and the grass eliminates the weeds for me. That's it in a nutshell, Weedy. You can do the same thing for your lawn."

"Well, I've been getting advice from the guys at the garden store, and they sold me some super weed killer. And I've been following the instructions on the label pretty well. But look at my yard — ugly as ever."

"I know, Weedy. I've been watching you. You see, I don't care how selective your weed killer is; when you spray it on your lawn the grass suffers some too, and that's why it's so sparse. And then if you don't really keep up with the job new weeds keep coming up, either from the seeds of the old weeds or from new seeds which are always blowing in on everybody's lawn."

"And that means your lawn too, right? So how come you don't get new weeds too, or even old weeds?"

"Because I keep my grass so healthy and thick that weeds don't stand a chance. You have so much bare space in your lawn that it's an open invitation to anything that wants to grow there. Sorry, Weedy, but that's how nature keeps our world green and beautiful."

"Are you telling me, Greeny, that those guys at the garden store have the wrong slant? After all, they're pros at this business and they learned their stuff in college. Both of them are horticulture majors, I found out."

"No, Weedy, I'm not telling you anything about those pros, though I'll say that pros in all fields make mistakes too. And sometimes these mistakes make money for them. I'd say that's good enough a reason for making mistakes, wouldn't you? Anyway, I'm just telling you what I think is the better way and the way I do my lawn.."

"You know, Greeny, I like your concept, and I'm going to do my lawn your way. Thanks for the advice."

"Good for you, Weedy. I've been wanting to wise you up ever since I moved here. Any time you have any more question, just ask, okay? But you've got the basic concept already, so I think in a few months you'll be happy with your new lawn."

"Well, Mr. Weedpatch did follow Mr. Greenlawn's advice and now he's got Mr. Greenlawn a bit perturbed, because he's always casting about innuendoes that his lawn is the prettiest on the block, if not in the whole town.

Lawn care is not the only field in which Mr. Greenlawn's principles apply. In fact our health can benefit in a very similar manner. If only more people would see their own mistakes the way Mr. Weedpatch did his, and take charge of their own lives....

CHAPTER SEVEN

BIG MEDI$IN

First let us define our subject. Who or what is Big Medi$in? It is not so much who as it is what it is, because the personal perpetrators are not easy to recognize. They operate mostly in the shadows and do not seek fame for their accomplishments. But their fruits are substantial and all too painfully effective and significant in the lives of the human race, especially in the U.S. of A., where the free enterprise system reigns supreme. "What" Big Medi$in is, is much more definitive, albeit also elusive to all but the comparative few who have attempted to understand it, either by force in self defense or for academic reasons. I happen to fall in both categories.

Big Medi$in for our purposes here is the attitude and modus operandi of the medical establishment in America, the spirit of self-enrichment, and its cause is human nature, an appreciation of the finer things of life, like a good education, impressive mansions, expensive automobiles, sleek yachts, life in a country club, and social status. All of these are very normal.

Though, as we have indicated, the "who" of Big Med are not very easy to identify, the organizations to which they belong, and from which they maintain their power through the advantages of unity and fiscal strategy, are not so nebulous, and in fact very conspicuous, or at least very, very significant and instrumental in the affairs of mankind.

Among the most active and aggressive of these organizations are the American Medical Association (AMA), the American pharmaceutical industry, and your own Food and Drug Administration (FDA). Collectively they are known by some as the Unholy Trinity. Not only do these mighty institutions work harmoniously within their own individual ranks; they cooperate admirably well with one another. And why not? It's no trick to work together when we have a common incentive. "You scratch my back and I'll scratch yours."

> "*There is a great deal of human nature in people.*"
> — Mark Twain

These three clubs are by no means the only ones belonging to what some refer to as the Medical Conspiracy. A few of the others are the America Cancer Society (ACS), the National Cancer Institute (NCI), the American Heart Association (AHA), and the insurance industry.

There are numerous others, but not all of them are strong, dyed-in-the-wool, active, aggressive members of the Conspiracy. Most are nebulously affiliated with the gang. And, again, it's human nature that brings these entities together in a common campaign. We all tend to foster conditions which feather our nests.

If human nature is at the base of this so-called conspiracy against the rest of us, it follows that as normal beings they should not be too severely criticized for being what they are. They are merely trying to make a "living" for themselves and their families. It's the American way, as they say. So in spite of where the chips fall as I try to shape my explanations, I hereby tell you that it is very much not my intent to condemn, or even derogate, our medicine men and women.

Such would not be at all constructive. But if I am to write a book to help you help yourself and attain what you bargained for, it is absolutely imperative that I "tell it like it is," or at least how I think it is after a few decades of pertinent study and experience. So I am trying to give you as clear a picture as I can to enable you to recognize what you are dealing with, or what you're up against, as you navigate your way toward glowing, robust health for yourself and family. In other words, if you would reach your destination do not try to change the sea; observe and study the tide and set your own sails accordingly.

The primary tool of Big Medi$in, if I had to name only one, is misinformation, some of it very direct and some in various degrees of subtlety. Some unhappy, disgruntled, frustrated patients, as well as some persons who have a strong propensity toward the well-being and happiness of their human family, characterize the misinformation as outright deceit and bold-faced lies. I am very sorry to have to agree with them, because numerous physicians and pharmacists, upstanding members of the medical orthodoxy, are unwarrantedly tainted by the attitudes and actions of the powers of the industry. Not only that; it pains me to observe anybody victimize anybody, especially in this realm where the stakes are sky-high. It is not at all an exaggeration to say that this human nature we speak of that is responsible for the attitude and modus operandi of mainstream medicine is responsible for horrendous measures of human suffering and millions of premature deaths. People die at 75 in what should be their prime of life, 30 or 40 years before their time, after years of unhappiness brought on by frustrating disease which our Creator did not design into our lives. Big Medi$in has conveniently forgotten the Oath of Father

Hippocrates while wantonly and defiantly violating Mother's beneficent laws.

" The pillars of truth and the pillars of freedom — they are the pillars of society."

— Henrik Ibsen

The manner in which Big Medi$in commits medicine is only half its crime. At every opportunity it attacks the practitioners, orthodox or alternative, who more altruistically adhere to the Hippocrates Oath and Mother's laws. It consistently opposes every attempt of the "quacks" to enhance true health. Thus far it has enjoyed a good measure of success, but the agents of truth are gradually gaining ground and reclaiming their rightful authority. More MDs are flying the coop. By promulgating the truth I am trying to hasten this process. Millions of the walking dead are crying for help but don't know where to find it. I'm trying to help show them the way.

"Why do you accuse the men and women of our most honored profession of such attitudes and actions? After all, they are among the best people in America." True, they are good people. They worked very hard to get where they are. But they are human, and as the saying goes, when money is on the table, all truth and compassion fly out the window. Have you noticed that I have not used the term "medical profession?" I use the term "medical industry" as a euphemism, because the "R" word is not polite, and I'm trying very hard to be kind to the American doctor, because he is also my brother and because he too is being exploited by Big Med, who panders to his innate human nature and creates for him such creature comforts and luxuries that are next to impossible to forego.

> "*He does not possess wealth that allows it to possess him.*"

— Benjamin Franklin

Before continuing, I want to be sure to acknowledge the merits and virtues of many conventional doctors and their conventional practices. In cases of traumatic injuries and certain emergencies, conventional is the only way to go. Not only that; conditions often develop where the patient tries his very utmost but simply cannot solve his problem. His symptoms are so unbearable that he is beside himself. Nature-oriented practitioners are nowhere conveniently nearby. He should obtain the services of an M.D. and of course also honor his own judgment in how he participates in his treatment. Many people go through life without needing the services of the medical orthodoxy. All I'm saying is that we should keep a firm hand on our physical and mental welfare and not go through life with our destiny in anybody else's hands, especially when we don't know what, why, and how those hands are doing to you.

Where Big Medi$in is concerned, there is very much to talk about, much more than cabbages and kings. I once agreed unequivocally and vehemently that America's capitalistic free-enterprise system was the very best political system in the world. Now, with more tough living under my belt, I'm not so sure. For many years I belonged to the National Republican Party, paying my dues and more. I was a true right-winger. Now I don't know what I am, except disillusioned.

The freedom which is at the very heart of our system allows and encourages the strong, the courageous, the intelligent, the immoral, the amoral, the privileged, to triumph over those who are not. I once subscribed to the validity of that philosophy too. In other words, the law of the jungle, catch-as-catch-can. That was the only way America can be strong and build character. But eventually I began to see that the people triumphed over had very little freedom to free themselves from the power of the triumphant. Nonetheless I still maintained some feeling that "survival of the fittest" was Mother's way and that we should abide by it. But high-powered philosophy can do only so much in the development of one's lifestyle, especially in the face of untenable conditions. For what good is a philosophically correct system if it kills people?

It is a popular notion that strength, courage, intelligence, and ability should be rewarded with the bounties of our world. But it is popular only among those of us who possess those qualities, and they are the ones who articulate that notion. The ones bereft of those qualities are innately incapable of articulating their views. And so they are still behind either the proverbial door or the proverbial eight-ball.

If the positive qualities may be considered innate, it hardly seems fair that they be counted as credits in the accounting, as they were already counted in the opening balance, and their possessors are not the ones who developed them. And what of some other qualities possessed by those of us who are not so generously endowed by fate: lack of opportunity, lack of native ability, physical weakness, mental retardation, lack of courage? Should these be counted as debits in the book of life? That doesn't seem fair either; their possessors came into this life already burdened by them and so are not at fault for them.

So how should the books be balanced? I don't really know; I'm asking questions now, not dispensing information. But I do know that we should all have equal opportunity. But our government seems to, indeed does, favor the ones already favorably endowed, increasing their advantages even more. And for understandable reasons: First, it is staffed by such people. Secondly, it is apparent that financial politics are the overriding factor. Morality does not come in for much consideration either. T.O. McCoye said something similar to what we said a few lines back: "When the dollar sign enters the field of health or religion, sincerity and love fade away." When there is no sincerity or love, truth is also absent, and therein lies the root of all the disagreement on the subject of health and disease. Because it behooves all of us to know the truth to the best of our ability, it seems sensible that we should make an effort to know whom to believe. It also seems sensible that the more credible informer is the one who is less influenced by the almighty dollar in his mutterings, not he who has an axe to grind, who is raking in the clams. Don't look at me, because 90 percent of all book writers lose money, so they say.

So what are the disadvantaged to do? In the field of health and disease they can band together and as a group participate in the law-making processes of our land. Sounds easy, but how does one little disadvantaged and frustrated patient go about banding together? His voice is but a whisper in a whirlwind. But all is not hopeless; far from hopeless. Others before him have already made that effort and are doing very well against great odds. Our disadvantaged patient is invited to join the National Health Federation, a very worthy and dedicated organization whose address is:

The National Health Federation
P.O. Box 688
Monrovia, CA 91016
Telephone (818) 357-2181

The goals of this organization are:
- To protect the individual's right to freedom of choice in health matters.
- To prevent and eradicate monopolies in the health field.
- To expose deficiencies and hazards of the orthodox health care system.
- To get facts on new developments in the health field.
- To receive updates on legal and legislative battles in the health freedom struggle.
- To provide educational materials for legislators and other government officials.
- To uphold individual health rights through legal action if necessary.
- To work for enactment of effective health freedom legislation.

Regular membership annual dues are $36. Seniors, $24; students, $24; foreign members, $48. Membership includes an exceedingly fine monthly magazine entitled Health Freedom News, in my estimation the very best health magazine I have ever seen, bar none. On even a purely selfish basis, this magazine makes it all worthwhile, giving the reader abundant thought-provoking information on health.

Membership in the Federation makes you a part of a humanitarian body without whom the poor patient (and the rich one too) would be in even a worse predicament than he is in now. Big Med is on a relentless program to usurp more and more of your freedom and money in the field of health and disease. Why do you think "health care" (disease care) is so outlandishly expensive, costing close to a trillion shimoleons annually? That's close to $4000 per person.

196

Why doesn't most health insurance pay for the less orthodox health treatments? Why does Big Med seem always to suppress and bad-mouth research and new knowledge in natural cancer treatments and force us to suffer the monstrously expensive, torturous and risky slash, poison, and burn protocol of the orthodoxy? Sorry; the three technical terms do not adequately describe the protocol. I know, because I've watched them kill my friends. Especially in view of this deplorable situation, I can't overstate the worthiness of the NHF and the worthwhileness of joining this group of people dedicated to health and, more important, freedom from tyranny.

> "*The only legitimate right to govern is an express grant of power from the governed.*"
>
> — William Henry Harrison.
> (Let us not continue to tacitly grant that power.)

Another thing you can do to protect yourself and family from the alleged tyranny of the powers is to learn all you can about Big Medi$in, the money-oriented industry you presently must put up with whenever you fall ill and even when you don't. This chapter will help you do that.

A third way is to learn all you can about your and your family's bodies and how to care for them. The chapters on Mother's Marvelous Machine and on Requisites For Health will help you do that. You will then be less dependent on entities whose services are more often than not of dubious value over all. When you learn how to cook you won't have to marry any old woman who comes along just so you can eat.

Complaints abound about medical malpractice by individual entities, but far too few people recognize the

197

profoundly damaging effects of the mostly unchallenged general concepts, attitudes, purpose, and actions of medicine as committed in the U.S. of A. To examine those concepts and attitudes is one of my major purposes, as the consequences of the alleged offenses are far more pervasive, encompassing, and devastating than all the cases of malpractice combined.

It is not the job of the American doctor to keep or make you well. It should be but it's not. His job is to placate you, to make you happy. So let's get out of the dark ages and out into the light of realty. You have two choices: (1) Get well and stay well or (2) Go to a conventional American doctor, stay sick, get sicker, and lose a goodly portion of your life savings. A paint job, no matter how high-tech the paint, simply will not do when your house is being blighted by termites and wet rot. In fact the paint may even provide a protective cover to allow the damage to proliferate.

If the doctor is not fulfilling our requirements for health, where's the shortcoming? Well, the patient is naive, remiss, and irresponsible in not knowing what he's getting for his health dollar, and the doctor is remiss in allowing the patient to bask in his own ignorance. But if a painter doesn't paint, he and his family don't eat. If a doctor doesn't push drugs, he and his family must be satisfied with a 24-foot sailboat, get stuck with a Buick, and perhaps must even drop out of the country club. What do you expect, anyway?

Conventional medicine has its place in society, and at appropriate times MDs can be godsends, and I appreciate them accordingly. What I don't appreciate about them is their refusal to approach health and disease realistically. In fact they don't approach health at all. They pander to the patients' ignorance, naivete, irresponsibility, and vulnerability. But I understand that they're human and have a right to love the finer things of life too. So I don't have the right to impose my standards on them. But that doesn't mean we have to go along with their schemes. If we do, it's our fault. Let them do their thing and let us do ours. To each his own.

So let us not criticize the doctor for not keeping us well. That is not his function, nor his intent. It is the function of the specialist in preventive medicine, the health consultant, writers of health books and articles, but ultimately, ourselves. If we seek the doctor's services unwisely, expecting him to do our job for us, we may as well hire a painter to repair the foundation of our house.

Salem Kirban, in his book "How to Keep Healthy and Happy by Fasting," says, "I am amazed that the American Medical Association has not seen to it that more books were written on fasting and its merits." How naive can one be? The poor soul also says, "...it (the AMA) should first devote more of its attention to the prevention of illness rather than to its treatment. ...Is that too radical a thought to project to the AMA?" Yes, yes, Brother Salem, it certainly is too radical a thought. Mr. Kirban would like to tell the AMA what business to be in. The AMA knows exactly what it wants to be in, and it has been highly successful at its business. See for yourself. Look at its economic and social standings.

Brother Salem is not alone in his naivete. Numerous proponents, and even exponents, of natural health still wonder when Big Med is going to learn the truth about health and disease. And even Dr. Arthur F. Coco, presumably a member of the AMA, has been holding his breath since he wrote his book "The Pulse Test" in 1956 as he waits for Big Med to adopt the pulse test as a diagnostic tool for allergies. Please, Dr. Coco, you should know that nobody gets rich counting pulses. Better give up.

Is American medicine a failure? If failure can be construed as "falling short of a goal" or "not succeeding in an attempt," then American medicine has not failed at all and in fact has been a resounding success, a glorious Horatio Alger story. See how well the M.D. lives; that is, if you can wheedle an invitation to board his yacht. Especially when his victim thinks he has benefited, success is complete. But Alexander the Great wasn't fooled. He said, "I die by the help of too many physicians."

It's no secret that Big Medi$in, through its political power, which in turn emanates from its economic power, which in turn emanates from patient money power, possesses and thoroughly exploits a humongous advantage over its patients, rich and poor. Advantage, you say? And here I thought medical treatment was supposed to be a partnership, a win-win effort.

The ancient Chinese doctor was paid to keep his patients well. If the patient got sick, the doctor didn't get paid, and also had to provide medicine at his own expense. Not so with the American doctor. Even if he kills his patient, which he often does, he still collects a huge bill from the survivors of the deceased (killed). Not only that; the M.D. enjoys a unique, god-like status. He may charge his patients whatever he damned well pleases, absolutely unhampered by law, and the patient or his survivor absolutely has to pay it or face legal consequences, as well as credit degradation.

Several years ago I went to see an eye, ear, nose, and throat specialist to get relief for a mild springtime allergy. (I should have known better.) One x-ray shot was taken of my head, though I don't know why. I was given a series of scratch tests and saw the doctor for just a very few minutes. The bill was $432.33.

A few months later I went to an endocrinologist. I gave his nurse a urine specimen and two vials of blood for laboratory analyses. I returned a few days later for consultation with the doctor and was told that I was in good shape. The bill was $633.

Another time I had surgery on my ankle to repair some torn ligaments. The nurses told me the operation required about two-and-a-half hours. I was hospitalized for two days. The surgeon's bill was $3600. The hospital's was also $3600. Let's give the surgeon another half-hour, to change his clothes and such. Now, was his time worth $1200 per hour??? My medical problem being non-systemic, I presume I did not require any heroic or extraordinary services, mainly only recuperation and a few "hospital meals." For $3600 I must have received some awfully expensive anesthetics.

Is it any wonder that we hear not-so-funny jokes like the following?

"What's the difference between a doctor and a bat?"

"I dunno. What?"

"One is a greedy blood-sucking rat and the other is a rodent who lives in a cave."

Yes, I go to doctors and hospitals too. But at least I learned a lot of good stuff, and that is what I'm trying to share with you.

Let's get back to the first blood sucker, the one who sucked my $433.32. His nurses were visibly embarrassed and told me he charges such high fees to everybody, but new patients pay more because they're charged an extra $100 for opening a new account. One of his former nurses personally told me this story: One day an old man came in

201

pretty sick and was duly examined by Dr. Blood. After that visit the doctor found out that the man didn't have any medical insurance. When the old man came in for his second visit the doctor said to the nurse, "Go out there and tell Mr. So-and-So that I cannot see him. And tell him he'd better get some insurance or he's going to die." The nurse said, "I can't tell him that." The doctor said, "It's your job. Go tell him." The nurse said, "Go tell him yourself. I quit." And she quit.

Dr. Blood's mansion is famous, because, as seemingly everybody knows, it looks like a hotel. He takes vacations often and reportedly has many animal heads hanging in his trophy room. As you can see, he's not very selective as to whose blood he takes.

It dismays me to read so often that other countries are increasingly adopting the American way of committing medicine. Of all nations, even China is doing it. American doctors and corporations are building clinics and hospitals in foreign lands, exporting Yankee ingenuity, as they say. I have a strong urge to fly over to these countries and yell to them, "Don't follow us! Quit while you're behind!"

The logic, or lack thereof, of the mass of American people on matters of medical treatment puzzles and frustrates the hell out of me. They know, or should know, because it is so obvious, that disease is the doctor's stock in trade, all he has to work with, and that health is his nemesis, the increase of which is inversely proportional to the profits of his business. And yet they continue to look on doctors as virtual gods, saviors of America's sick. We must remember that haloes and angels' wings are not issued with medical diplomas and that doctors are still human beings like the rest of us. No, I didn't say inhumane beings.

Yet most Americans, even in matters of life and death, trust their doctors implicitly. Even when the patient disagrees with his doctor, he seems to say, "You're the doctor; you know best." Poppycock! Does our faithful patient really trust his doctor that much or is it that he lacks faith in himself and his own knowledge? I think it's more the latter, for I utterly fail to find any reason for anybody's believing all those illogical pronouncements of the medical establishment. I see axes in their hands and they want to use my grindstone. Sadly, even the educated patients, the PhDs among us, seem addicted to this unwarranted dependence on someone else. Call it a cop-out if you wish. I do.

To these insecure souls I say: Educate yourselves. There are numerous good books and magazine articles written by health researchers who have no axes to grind, who are not directly dependent for their livelihood on whether you opt for surgery, chemotherapy, radiation, or nutritive therapy. You should at least cut these disinterested parties in on your decision making. I remind you that the "Health Freedom News," the monthly magazine of the National Health Federation, is a splendid source of help. I just want you to at least contemplate who and what will help you and of whom and what to be wary. In other words, take charge of your own destiny. Don't depend on anybody unwarrantedly. Don't even swallow what I feed you without first tasting and chewing it.

You are the foremost specialist on your own life and health. Participate with your doctor. If he seems to have failed you, it may not be entirely his shortcoming. Perhaps you have neglected to do your part of the job. He can't go with you to the grocery store. He can't chase you to bed early. He can't go jogging with you. He can't philosophize for you. If you expect to be healthy you must do things for yourself.

Let me emphasize that there are many fine MDs. When I say fine I mean fine for the patient, not necessarily for the medical industry. Two that come to mind immediately are Dr. Jonathan V. Wright and Dr. Stuart M. Berger. I can't help thinking also of Dr. Clarence Farrar, now retired, who practiced in Manchester, Tennessee, my present home town. "Dr. Clarence," a good old-fashioned doctor who practiced good old conventional medicine as it was practiced before the medical gold rush, was very obviously concerned first and foremost for the patient. It wasn't long ago that he was active, but alternative medicine had not yet reached, and still hasn't reached, this small town of less than 8000. This is not to say the gold rush hadn't arrived in Manchester yet; it certainly had and of course is still here. But from what I have seen and heard of Dr. Clarence, he was true blue and never took advantage of these money-grubbing times.

Dr. Wright learned his medicine at Harvard and at the University of Michigan Medical School but has graduated into the wholistic mode of practice. He wrote a fine book entitled "Dr. Wright's Book of Nutritive Therapy," Rodale Press. Dr. Berger studied at Tufts University, a stronghold of preventive medicine, and at the Harvard School of Public Health. His book "What Your Doctor Didn't Learn in Medical School," William Morrow & Co., also is very good reading.

Obviously, both Drs. Wright and Berger have foregone the luxury and comfort of the establishment, but leaving the club is not free. There's an exit charge, especially if the departing member asserts himself in the wrong direction. The moment he does something of substance which is not in accord with the club's objectives, brother, he's asking for it. Especially if his assertions threaten to lower the lifestyles of the loyal members, like pulling one of their yachts out of the marina, well, what should you expect? On the morning of May 6, 1992, just before opening time, Dr. Wright's Tahoma Clinic in Kent, Washington, was raided by about twenty men from the FDA and the Kent Police Department. Reportedly they broke through the doors by kicking and with a sledgehammer. They entered by three entrances simultaneously with guns drawn and pointed at the dumbfounded staff. One staff member was physically injured. The entire contents of the building were hauled away.

Now, what crime was Dr. Wright accused of to deserve such ignominious treatment? He treated his patients with a natural adrenal cortical extract (ACE), a form of the drug with a record of generations of safe and effective use, even by mainstream physicians. What was so wrong about that? Well, a few years before that, our drug merchants developed a synthetic form of the drug and, by means of their usual medical politics, are now making more profits off the synthetic form than from the natural, which of course they no longer market. So now the natural form is no longer on the FDA's list of approved drugs, and any use of it is in direct competition with the man-made drug. It was strongly rumored that our then-President had heavy interests in one of the pharmaceutical icons.

One doctor's use of the Real McCoy of course isn't serious competition, but all the other stubborn mavericks had better observe the rules and conform. So the Tahoma Raid of 1992 stands as a shining example of how The Boys frown on the antics of upstart physicians. Not only should they refrain from using natural medicines; they should also refrain from using any simple, pragmatic, inexpensive remedy which will make people well. Like, "You don't need to bolster your diet with supplements. That's a bunch of superstition designed to take your money from you." Or, "Don't believe those quacks. Diet has nothing to do with your health." Who are the quacks? Who is taking your money by the billions and depleting your life savings? Medical costs are now so extreme that they are now ludicrously a very major factor in the terms of occupational employment. A company manufactures automobile tires but it also must finance its employees' health. Funny?

We already know that Big Medi$in is doing extremely well. But is it doing good? Doing good for whom? Or is it doing harm? Let's look at a few statistics.

In 1929 America spent $3 billion on health; in 1960, $26 billion. Today, close to a trillion dollars annually trying to keep well, and yet in comparison with other nations rank about 16th in longevity and 27th in health. Of the 22 most advanced western nations only Portugal is sicker than we are.

One of every two Americans can expect some day to enter a nursing home, the cost of which now averages some $30,000 annually. One of every three of us will some day contract cancer, and half of these will each pay $100,000 to die after terrible suffering.

If we do not stop this juggernaut of a trend, by the year 2000 we will spend about $1.5 trillion annually trying to keep half-well, which will probably be a more difficult task by then. Hey! As Edgar Taft Bensten said, "A trillion here, a trillion there, pretty soon we're talking big money." The difficulty will be exacerbated by the poverty foisted on us by the greed and stupidity of our nation's leaders, who, by the way, reside in the same elite enclave with Big Medi$in.

Overhaul our medical system and we can pay off the national debt in a few years, plus save a couple hundred billion dollars in interest annually. (Incidentally, today we're paying almost exactly a billion a day in interest.) A wild-eyed dream? Not at all. Even spectacularly successful revolutions look wild-eyed at first. Stop that humongous torrent of dollars draining into the medical rathole and the job is well on its way to reality. Then again, I guess it is a wild-eyed dream.

The FDA appears not a whit concerned (Why should it be?) about alcohol, tobacco, caffeine, and other legal drugs, and yet for decades has fought every attempt at health that comes along, including the administration of natural nutritive therapy for cancer and other maladies, despite the undeniable successes of that therapeutic discipline even in numerous terminal cases. It has treated many beneficent medical clinics like criminals and has forced them across our national boundaries. And ironically, all of this unfair, unethical, and unconstitutional activity is being perpetrated with money from the people, the very ones who are grossly injured by the political shenanigans of our government agencies and other special interests.

Big Medi$in has fought health for as long as I can remember, and now cancer is the leading killer of American children. I must wonder how many of our children are destined for the human scrap pile. Cancer or not, they appear headed for a rough time anyway.

Medical knowledge in America is purported to have increased some 40-to 50-fold since 1960, and yet in the same period the rate of cancer has doubled. Did this happen in spite of American medicine or because of it? Whether in spite of or because, it has been one big fiasco. Since 1900 our life expectancy has increased by just a few years, and the increase was due mostly to improvement in the rate of infant mortality. The record for adults is unspectacular at best, despite our abundant knowledge and huge expenditures.

It should be obvious from the foregoing that Big Medi$in is making and keeping America sicker with every shot of legal drugs. A friend told me she was taking 16 different prescription drugs simultaneously and doesn't understand why she is always sick. She also told me that the monthly out-of-pocket cost of prescription drugs for the two of them was between $200 and $300. And Medicare doesn't pay for drugs. Mercy! More recently this same friend was rushed by ambulance to the hospital with a heart attack, and one of her drugs was determined to be the cause. Another case of iatrogenic injury. She nevertheless had to pay for the "professional services rendered."

My mother suddenly became very ill. Everything seemed to be wrong with her. She was weak and nervous. Her mind was that of a child. My sisters and I wondered how senility had got the best of her so abruptly, as she had always been a lively, intelligent woman with a keen sense of humor. Her doctor couldn't figure her out either and finally suggested we put her in a nursing home, which we reluctantly did, sorrowfully wondering whether it was a permanent move. Poor Mom was a zombie. But despite her fuzzy state of mind, one day she said, "I think this medicine is what's making me sick. I'm going to stop taking it for a while. She did stop taking it and, wonder of wonders, she felt much better almost immediately. In a very few days we took her home. You guessed it. She resumed her active life and never got that sick again until her last days.

A few years ago a fairly well known hospital killed five of my close friends with chemotherapy within a period of two months. Especially ironic was that at least four of them entered the hospital thoroughly ambulatory and from outward appearances, the way they walked and talked, were in very normal condition. Only their malignancies belied their demeanor. They certainly did not look like terminal cases to me, and I have no way of knowing whether they would have survived without chemotherapy, but I can say for a certainty that my friends were killed in that hospital. Nobody dies that fast on his own.

> *"It is forbidden to kill; therefore all murderers are punished unless they kill in large numbers."*
>
> — Voltaire

That hospital also employs hyperthermia in the treatment of cancer, a procedure which gradually raises the patient's body temperature to 107.6 degrees, holds it there for an hour, and then brings it back down to normal. One patient there had had 14 such treatments at $8000 per. When I talked with him he had already paid $112,000, because his insurance company didn't cover hyperthermia. (And you know why.) One patient's husband who seemed to know what was what, obviously driven by desperation, presumed to talk to the owner of the hospital in protest of the unreasonably high cost of the treatment. According to him, he pushed the owner until he got the price down to $3000. But be consoled; I don't think anybody lost money because of the reduction in price.

The average charges at this hospital seemed to be very close to $1500 per day. One husband told me that his wife's charges over several weeks averaged over $1600 per day. Well, what do you think hospitals are for, anyway?

This benevolent institution ("We care.") is good for more exciting stories, but I've had enough of them, thank you.

Do you think $1500 per day is unreasonable? Well, be consoled again. A friend of mine took his son, who had muscular dystrophy, to a hospital at 8 a.m. The doctors there, feeling that the boy needed more specialized attention, instructed the father to take the boy to another hospital, in Nashville, about 76 miles away. The father drove his son there through city traffic, got through the medical consultation, and drove back, arriving at noon. It was then that I saw him, and he was very visibly still in shock, seemingly trying to shake himself out of a bad dream. The hospital in Nashville, he told me, had charged him $15,000 for that short visit.

If you stole something, say ten dollars, and got caught by the law, you'd be in trouble. If you did it by force, say with a gun, you'd be in big trouble. And if somebody got killed in the robbery, you'd really be in trouble.

But when a member of the Unholy Trinity robs somebody by force, even when somebody dies in the process, no sweat. Not only no sweat; the robber gets the money anyway, anything he wants, for the crime. And, brother, the estate of the victim had better pay up, or else. And the perpetrator goes his merry way without missing a beat, still enjoying the respect and gratitude of everyone, including the law.

Does something smell funny here? What the hell is the difference between these two types of robbery? It's not the type of robbery that's important here; it is the who of the robbery that determines whether it's a crime or a humanitarian service. In other words, you must be a member of the gang to enjoy impunity and the privilege of determining for and by yourself the amount of the heist.

I don't pretend to know just how this conspiracy works, but I do know that it is a corrupt country which not only allows such a racket to persist but also honors it. Should we wonder why we're in such a sorry state of decay?

> "*Those who commit injustice bear the greatest burden.*"
> — Hosea Balboa. Oh?

Every big city in America has several huge impressive hospitals. Some of them are downright awesome and spectacularly appointed. The casual observer probably thinks, "What a marvel! How fortunate we are to have these beautiful fine facilities to take care of our health!" Even I marvel at these high-tech glamorous edifices. But after regaining my perspective I say to myself, "What a crying pity that we need all these super-expensive facilities, not so much because of the expense of the structures, equipment, salaries, and what-not, but more because we need them so badly. We have been made to need them. Within these walls has been installed a self-regenerating business that keeps the populace in a recycling pattern. Is it any wonder that a few years ago a hospital corporation was the most profitable business in America that year?

In 1989 deaths due to prescription drugs numbered 160,000, and we have good reason to believe that in the years since, the number has risen. Can you believe that prescription drugs kill three times more people in one year than the American men and women killed in ten years in Vietnam amid the bombs, bullets, mines, and grenades? To add insult and more injury to the injury of death, probably every death had to be paid for by the survivors. Evidently the magic bullets are somewhat more effective than regular bullets. Aha! Here's a super suggestion for the next war: Open up American hospitals behind enemy lines.

211

It is roughly estimated that in 1989 there were 10,000 drugs on the American market and 2.4 billion prescriptions were written. Will someone please tell me, if drugs are so effective why do we need 10,000? After the first twenty-five, wouldn't one think we had enough?

In 1995 about 240,000 American women were afflicted with breast cancer, and about 60,000 of them died. That breaks down to 1200 per state, which further reduces to 23 per state per week. Simply put, one of our precious women dies of breast cancer every nine minutes. And that's from breast cancer alone. An untenable situation, but what can we do about it? Find a cure for cancer? That's a lot of bull and our educated people know it. We can't poison the body to health. This freedom in America to make money by hook or crook has gone much too far. This freedom is at the great expense of the freedom of millions of victims. And freedom is the right of every American, rich or poor, strong or weak. Huh? Oh. I guess I'm being naive again.

The "National Enquirer" a few years ago estimated that 4,500,000 patients were poisoned annually by prescription drugs badly enough to be sent to the hospital. The Rodale Press reported that 200,000 Americans die each year at the hands of doctors. That is called iatrogenic injury, and it's derived from the Latin "iatro," meaning doctor, and "gen," meaning produced by. The figures just quoted, remember, are from a few years back. Given the trends in medicine, you can guess pretty well what the figures are now.

While marveling at the wonders of American medicine, bear in mind that natural nutritive therapy for cancer is illegal in the U.S. of A. We've come a long way, Baby, since the days we founded this country in respect to God our Creator.

In 1973 the Chevra Kadish, the Jewish burial organization, was reported as saying that the number of burials performed by them had dropped 60 percent since the beginning of a doctors' strike. A similar reduction had occurred during a doctors' strike there in 1953. Israel doesn't have a monopoly on these interesting stories. During a five-week doctors' strike in Los Angeles the death rate dropped below "normal." After the strike the rate rose above normal.

Dr. Hardin B. Jones of the University of California produced statistics to show that cancer patients who undergo the conventional treatments live an average of three more years after the treatments. Those who decline the conventional treatments live an average of 12.5 more years.

A 1986 article states: "The average malpractice insurance cost for specialists on the West Coast is now considerably higher than the average income: $36,000 yearly! By way of contrast, malpractice insurance for alternative practitioners, particularly nutritionists, runs less that $200 annually." Is this a reflection on trustworthiness?

According to a Boston University report: "The average hospital patient receives nine to ten drugs during his stay, and about 30 percent of all hospital patients suffer at least one bad reaction to drugs during their stay."

Angiograms are notoriously inaccurate, and 90 percent of them are unnecessary. Balloon angioplasty carries a two-to-seven percent death rate. Thirty-five percent of the cleared blockages return for re-opening within six months. About five percent of all bypass operations are fatal, whereas the death rate is less than two percent for the disease itself. Fourteen thousand to 28,000 are killed annually by bypass operations. Ironically, several available alternative remedies, much safer and much less expensive, have been obstructed

213

by means of non-coverage by insurance. Listen. Nobody said they were stupid.

Let me quote you some drug prices I have personally observed recently: Seventy capsules of Zovirax, $89. A 2-ounce tube of Zostrix cream; active ingredient, Capsaicin 0.025 percent. That's .002 ounce or 0.0142 gram of the active ingredient, and the price of the 2-ounce tube was $23. How do you like this one? I don't recall what the medicine was but it was 60 tablets for $255. No comment.

The American Cancer Society was founded in 1913, coincidentally the same year in which the Federal Reserve Board was sneaked in on us suckers. Now, 84 years later, cancer is rampaging worse than ever. In fact it's about ten times worse. Don't you think it's about time to give up on the project? Are you kidding? Things are moving along just copasetically. Research to find a cure is much more lucrative than finding one. The ACS is legally a non-profit organization because its fat salaries are technically expenses rather that profit. Isn't that neat? About 56 percent of the $160 million-or-so given them by the concerned and trusting public annually goes for salaries and other administrative expenses. About 30 percent goes for researching a cure for cancer, not by themselves, but subbed out to other researchers. Now, these subcontractors have administrative expenses too; so just how much money actually goes for research? It gives me great comfort to know that out of every heartfelt dollar you give to the ACS, at least 15 cents goes to cancer research. And of course it takes money to fight the quacks, the ones who threaten to really find cures and also those who are too successful in helping Mother prevent and cure cancer. The almighty dollar which you give to the ACS every year has been very instrumental in forcing some very sincere and successful cancer clinics to seek refuge in Mexico and the Caribbean Islands. Some undeniably sincere and dignified scientists have had the rug pulled out from under their very promising projects. Here are just a few of them: (1) Dr. Andrew C. Ivy of the University of Chicago, who was eminently respected by his colleagues until his potentially successful Kriebiozen showed too much potential. A documented fact is that a high official of the AMA secretly tried to get himself cut in on the marketing of Kriebiozen. When he was refused access to the new substance, he said, "You'll rue this day." And that was the end of Kriebiozen and the fame of Dr. Ivy, whose name now languishes in comparative obscurity behind the proverbial eight-ball. (2) Dr. Ernst Kriebs, the developer of laetrile. Only after years of fighting by freedom-loving entities, including the National Health Federation, laetrile is now available legally in this great freedom-loving nation. (3) Harry Hoxey, whose clinic was outlawed in our country and now operates in Mexico. I have no authoritative opinion on the Hoxey Clinic, but I do know that it is still very popular, having just recently erected a new impressive building to house its operations. I also know that its methods are wholistic and uses natural substances. Big Medi$in was highly successful in defaming the late Mr. Hoxey, for to this day many people regard the Hoxey people as quacks. My impression from my studies is that the Hoxey Clinic is true blue. (4) Dr. Max Gerson. I could write a whole book on this man. Originally from Austria, he made a fine gift of himself to our country when he came here, only to have the gift trashed by Big Medi$in. We'll talk about this great man a bit later on, but for now suffice it say that no less a celebrity than the late Dr. Albert Schweitzer referred to Max Gerson as the greatest genius in the history of medicine.

How is it that doctors continue to charge more and more for their disservices and patients still crowd their waiting rooms? Because people are getting sicker and sicker. And people are getting sicker and sicker because their lack of knowledge, fostered by Big Med, leaves them no choice but to keep returning to the doctors' offices.

When asked whether they feared the cost of health care, one percent of the Japanese interrogated said yes, as did two percent of the British, three percent of the Germans, five percent of the Canadians, and 27 percent of the Americans. Despite Medicare, many Americans worry that they will be wiped out if they need to go to a nursing home. They are also scared of the specter of having to regularly pay for drugs. And remember that despite all the money we spend for health we still rank 27th in health internationally.

I don't know how the following information slipped out of their inner sanctums, but according to JAMA, the Journal of the AMA, of all the former smokers questioned, only 3.6 percent said that their doctors had helped them quit. There are still 50,000,000 smokers in the U.S., and the huge majority of them would like to quit. Anti-smoking prescription drugs are not reimbursable by most insurance companies, and for good reason: One-fourth of the nation's health care costs are spent on tobacco-related illnesses. One of six deaths is caused by smoking. (Too bad. There goes one golden goose.) I don't have to tell you that Big Med is very much involved in the insurance business. Only recently has Big Med finally started to admit that smoking is somewhat detrimental to health, and only because it can no longer put the cat back into the bag. One doctor recommended in print that one should try to limit tobacco consumption to only one pack a day. It wasn't too many years ago that doctors advertised cigarettes in full-page colorful ads in the big magazines and newspapers, and were paid for their endorsements by the tobacco companies.

Many years ago as a young man I noticed that Big Medi$in, despite its appropriate position in society, never dispensed beneficial health information until and unless forced to by public knowledge. When just about everybody had been convinced of a health fact by other entities, that's when Medi$in jumped on the band wagon by way of the tailgate, bullied its way with its prestige and financial power into the driver's seat, and usurped the credit by echoing what the quacks had been recommending for the last half-century. Now we're hearing more often, "The doctor says we shouldn't be smoking." Oh, this fascinating world of competition and strategy.

Here's the system: Whenever health-enhancing information is promulgated by the "quacks," Medi$in ignores it as long as it can, in effect partially negating it with its silence and its prestige. When the information is out on the streets and can be ignored no longer, Medi$in contradicts and ridicules it. When the contradiction and ridicule begin to look silly and the public is now wise to the facts, they jump on the band wagon with horns blowing and streamers streaming and claim the great new discovery as their very own. Tobacco has completed the cycle, having taken close to a century to do it. Currently, the name of the American Cancer Society graces the packaging of quit-smoking transdermal patches. Hah! Exceptionally profitable items take longer than most. Diet is just now entering the final stage of the system. It has taken, oh, so long to get here. Both these items were in the first stage before I was born in 1919. Look back and see if you can recognize the strategy at work.

Now, don't think for a moment they have completely knuckled under on smoking and diet. They still advise their patients to cut down on cigarettes. Remember the MD who advised smoking no more than one pack a day? And they're still fighting diet pretty hard, even with their backs to a corner. In fact many of the gang are still trying to ignore the problem. Good luck, boys! A recent magazine article by an MD announced that research has revealed that diet has a significant effect on health, perhaps as much as 30 percent. Really? That much? Doctors are such fascinating people.

"It is difficult to make a man understand something when his salary depends on his not understanding it."
— Upton Sinclair

What's so wrong with our health care system? First, it's not a health care system at all. It's a disease-propagation and merchandising system, inspired by all the high-powered strategy of Madison Avenue. It is one of the most successful industries in the world, raking in billions of dollars and in return broadcasting disease and misery to its faithful customers. This disease and misery, being part of the cycle, are returned to the medical factory for reprocessing. The paying customers are drugged into feeling well and released to incubate more fresh raw material for the factories. On and on it goes, ad nauseum...

"Two wrongs do not make a right."
— English proverb.
(Poisoning your body and robbing your bank account do not make you healthy.)

218

By the way, if you're beginning to feel I'm a know-it-all, I'll have to admit to something: I have no conclusive evidence that Big Medi$in is in any way affiliated with the surreptitious New World Order.

> *"As long as the world shall last, there will be wrongs, and if no man objected and no man rebelled, those wrongs would last forever."*
> — Clarence Darrow

> *"Rebellion against tyrants is obedience to God."*
> — Benjamin Franklin

As we have said, Big Medi$in has its place in society. (Does it!) It's not so much what it does, how it does it, and how much money they take from us that's doing us patients in; it's more the attitude of us patients that causes us to depend so much on the doctors that we feel we can abuse our bodies with impunity. This attitude can be entertained only so long. If we live long enough, the day will come when we will have to change it.

In 1996 two major airline crashes hit the news. First a ValuJet plane went down in the Florida Everglades. Then TWA Flight 800 exploded in mid-air and crashed off Long Island. Both of these tragedies of course rocked the nation and remained in the news for months. Huge amounts of money and human effort were spent on trying to fathom the causes of these misfortunes, not to mention the unfathomable depths of human suffering on the parts of the victims and survivors. The aftermath of the ValuJet crash in the Everglades entailed almost impossible human efforts as divers searched for remnants of the wreckage far below the surface in murky water with virtually zero visibility. The cause of the TWA crash was also extremely puzzling, and at this time, more than a year later, the parties involved are still working very hard on the puzzle.

I am extremely grateful that we live in a country that cares this much about our fellow men, women, and children. After all, it's not every day that about 400 people lose their lives within a span of a few weeks.

No, this doesn't happen every day. What does happen every day is that the number of people who die of heart disease is large enough to fill about a dozen jumbo jets. Yes more than a million people die of heart disease every year. But are we as concerned and grieved by these deaths as we are over those two airplane crashes? I'm afraid not. And why not? It seems people are apathetic about these deaths, feeling perhaps that nothing more can be done to prevent them, that the supposed stewards of our health are already doing everything possible for us. But the fact is that much more can be done to prevent heart disease. And I do mean very much more. So why aren't the doctors doing it? If there's something we can do to keep ourselves healthy, why aren't we doing it? Why don't the doctors teach us how to be healthy? After all, doesn't "doctor" mean "teacher?" Are you kidding? They are not stupid. Actually, loads of good information are floating around in our country, but most of us are ignoring it, and for several reasons. Hot dogs, chips, ice cream, and coke are just too enjoyable. Exercise is too much of a drag. But the most potent deterrent to our health is the attitude instilled in us by Big Medi$in. But why should Big Med try to teach us? After all, it's not their job anymore. Besides, as I've said, they're not stupid. As long as we keep going back to them seeking the same old treatment, they'll give it to us. And do they give it to us! That's their job.

We ourselves are mostly to blame. We're passing the buck. Ultimately it is our job to care for ourselves and our families. So let's do our job and do it right. Let's regain the dignity of skippering our own ship, of being the master of our lives. If you feel being a health nut is too much of a drag, go visit a nursing home soon and think about it again.

Let's bring the pieces together and try to simplify our assessment of mainstream American medicine.

Notwithstanding all I've said about Big Medi$in, doctors are high-level people, capable, intelligent, hard-working. They do heroic things for their patients, like saving countless lives. They have earned the respect and gratitude of their patients. I myself have often felt profoundly grateful to my doctors.

I wish I could right here end this characterization of the American doctor, but such would not be appropriate, for there is much more to be considered regarding the subject. Sad to say, the heroics of Big Med, when examined in the light of reality, lose some of their net worth. Look back on your own encounters with your doctors and you will realize that much, very much, of the services they render merely compensates for adverse results of their treatment. And this is true of even the best and most skilled of them. This is inevitable, because the practice of conventional medicine is saturated with harmful effects. The methods and materials used are by and large inimical to the benevolent natural processes of Mother's Marvelous Machine. Drugs do incalculable damage to our bodies. Their intended benefits are superficial and temporary while their side effects are so profound as to be a major bane to the human race. In fact, "side effects" are in reality often primary effects. Then there are the x-rays, other forms of radiation, drastic chemicals, unnecessary surgery including the removal of valuable organs. What ever happened to Father Hippocrates' "First do no harm"?

Notice that a very huge proportion of the physical suffering in hospitals is the result of "complications" and not the original problem. These unexpected setbacks are all but inevitable given the drastic nature of the materials used to get us "well." And, just as absurdly, a huge proportion of the astronomical financial cost is also attributable to these complications.

Ironically, and obviously illogically, the more unsuccessfully a regular doctor treats his patient, the more compensatory work he creates for himself, and the more he is financially compensated for his failures. What a lovely business to be in, where one is handsomely rewarded for his failures, even fatal ones, as well as for the sure-fire side effects of his dangerous symptom-relieving drugs. One doctor killed my father by a stupid and stubborn mistake!

What a considerable difference there is between the respective practices and materials employed by MDs and alternative practitioners. The alternatives by and large attempt to help their patients by improving their health in accordance with Mother Nature's laws while Big Medi$in and true health are mutually antithetical.

We have looked at the proverbial tip of the iceburg, which is solidly supported by a formidable structure of misinformation and misdirection. This distortion of truth by Big Med is perhaps more damaging than the actual practice of its members, for we poor lemmings fall for their stuff and use it as a guiding light to determine our way of life and health. And what a way it is, compared to what it could and should be.

So you can see that Big Med pushes its cause not only in their offices, clinics, and hospitals, but also by proxy, using us victims as their agents.

Again, conventional doctors are high-level people. It is regretfully ironical and pitiable that such talent as they possess should be used for a purpose other than the ostensible. Oh well, they have chosen their way of life and have the right to operate their business as profitably as they can. It's the American way, after all.

Notwithstanding his lofty station in the society of planet Earth, notwithstanding the adulation heaped upon him by his trusting and hapless patients, if he continues to follow the addicting flute of his Pied Piper of Prosperity, if he continues to remain ignorant of the true workings of Mother's Marvelous Machine, if he continues to knowingly violate her laws, if he continues to pander to the ignorance and weaknesses of the less fortunate among us, the typical American doctor will continue to be doomed to a career of unconscionable and tragic disservice to his human siblings, his brothers and sisters in the family of our benevolent Creator. That's how it is. Amen.

Oh well, the American conventional doctors have chosen their way of life and have the right to operate their business as profitably as they can. It's the American way, after all.

But remember, you have rights too, a choice, and a God-given brain. Take charge!

Before leaving this subject let us take a look at the practitioners in the alternative disciplines of medicine and health. I once thought they were a far different breed of humanity from the MDs. They're not. They're human too, with human desires and ambitions. I like their approaches to health much better than conventional medicine, hands down in fact, but many of them also look on their patients as cash cows. So, as far as money is concerned, shifting over to an alternative doctor is not the same as jumping out of the frying pan onto the stovetop. You may be jumping into another frying pan, because there's not much stovetop area left these days. It seems everybody's got his frying pan out and ready to catch anybody who dares jump.

Do not patronize an alternative doctor because your MD is robbing you, is greedy, or is irresponsible. Everybody's human, and these days more people seem to be greedy and irresponsible. The best protection you have against other human beings is to be your own authority, your own master. Then you can also be your own best doctor. Develop your own health practice and go to the professionals only when you must. Not only will you be healthier, you will also be comparatively free.

But to be your own doctor you must know what to do, not so much for your ailments but for your health. For when you're healthy you won't get sick. The chapter on health can help you keep healthy. Your public library has many good health books. Study them.

Alternative medicine is not simply alternative medicine. It comprises several widely varying disciplines, some of which are naturopathy, chiropractic, homeopathy, neuromuscular massage, shiatsu, physical therapy, acupuncture, reflexology, Christian Science, bio-magnetic touch, not to mention numerous less prominent ones. Almost all of them are beneficial, because they evolved mostly from creative people's minds and not from Madison Avenue. Forget osteopathy; it's not an alternative anymore. It has capitulated to Big Medi$in and is now part of it.

Obviously it would require another book to explain all these methods; so we'll leave it at that. But I will say that naturopathy is one of my favorites, and that is because, as I understand it, it tends to treat the whole body by Mother's laws and is not overly concerned about specific symptoms.

Whatever alternative practice you prefer, if it respects Mother and doesn't shoot you full of drugs, it's bound to be better than Big Medi$in.

If you have kept current on health information, you probably know that researchers in true health have added much dramatic information of late. If you have not, and health is important to you, try to keep up with these new developments. Some of them are truly fascinating — and beneficial.

CHAPTER EIGHT

REQUISITES FOR HEALTH

If you would be truly healthy you will have to follow just about all the advice on the following pages. But that is not my intent. The health measures I suggest are fairly stringent, but that doesn't mean you must do everything I suggest. However you feel about my thoughts, don't let me discourage you. Take from these pages what you want and disregard what you don't. Frankly, my wish is that you become and remain fairly healthy, free enough of disease to afford you a future unhampered by handicapping conditions. For there are other components of life to enjoy in addition to a super-healthy body. But if you aspire to become the paragon of health in addition to having a super-fulfilling life, so much the better.

You don't have to feel glowingly good all the time. By saying this I am not trying to lower your standards of excellence. You see, feeling bad is very much a part of health. It goes with the process of restoring your homeostasis, because at those times your body, with Mother's help, is busy in its work of purging itself of undesirable factors. And that's good, isn't it? Back in the chapter "Quid Pro Quo," Howard Sharp explained to Belle how the common cold restores health to the body and in fact appears to decrease a person's chances of contracting cancer and other chronic "diseases." This is why I say you don't have to sacrifice too many of life's pleasures in order to enjoy good health with a clear conscience. Be reasonably fair with Mother and she'll be more than fair with you.

According to Carl Jung, "The afternoon of life must also have a significance of its own and cannot be merely a pitiful appendage of life's morning." To this I add, "If it's to be, it's up to me." Also remember that today is the first day of the rest of your life. No matter what your condition is today, you can be a new person in a very few months. Your body is magnanimously forgiving and renews itself constantly. But the quality of the renewal depends almost wholly on what help you give it. If you're going to renew anyway, why not renew with quality material?

It is all too common to see health seekers taper off and give up on their program, and I think the reason is that they don't see and feel results soon enough. And that's understandable. "I do all these nice things for my health and I still feel bad. In fact I feel worse." If this is the way you feel about the results of your efforts, it's because you don't fully understand that at such times your body is doing its work of restoring your homeostasis, and work usually involves some effort and discomfort, much as a weekend of housecleaning involves getting tired and perhaps some sore muscles and joints. But you now have a clean house. You may want to go back and listen in as Howard explains to Belle how this mechanism works.

It's ironic that one should give up on his program just when he's beginning to get the results he's been working for. Please believe me, if you persevere results will come. If you keep shoveling dirt into the hole, though at first you may not see results, the hole will fill up. Faith and perseverance will see you through.

I take care of my health so that I may enjoy some vices with impunity and a clear conscience. I try to maintain a positive advantage big enough that the next breeze won't bowl me over. I may be durable enough to stand against even a hurricane.

Life is to be lived and enjoyed. But you cannot really enjoy it without real health. So good old Socrates was pretty much on the ball when he advocated moderation in all things. He wasn't called a philosopher for nothing.

What good is a sleek ship in tip-top condition if it never goes to sea? So go out to sea now and then. But first be sure your ship is seaworthy, and give it a tune-up when you return. Eat a little piece of pink-frosted cake at your daughter's wedding. Have a beer with an old friend, if that's what you want to do. You'll know you're in good shape. Conserve your disciplinary efforts for where they will count for the most benefits.

But don't be like Ben. It was said of him: "Ben spent most of his money on women and booze. The rest he wasted."

But good health is not everybody's aspiration. Some people actually enjoy ill health, even while not realizing it. Some don't especially enjoy ill health but tolerate it as a condition of the kind of life they choose to live. As for me, sickness makes me extremely unhappy. If you're like me, let's consider a very simple concept: If you don't want to be sick you must be healthy. Yes, I know that sounds overly simplistic and flippant. But there are conditions that tend to keep that simple concept out of our clear view. First, some of us just don't care that much about it. And that's okay; it's not my calling to examine their philosophy. But I think the most influential factor that keeps our attitude nebulous and indifferent is the subtle but effective conspiracy of misdirection and misinformation foisted on us by Big Medi$in. It's not important that the word "doctor" derives from the Latin word meaning "teacher." Whatever useful information we have learned about health and disease we have wrested from life despite the machinations of Big Med. This book is written in an effort to overcome the stifling effects of these conditions.

To those brave and complacent souls who don't give a toot about health, let me say this: So many old, and not so old, people say, "Old age is such a horrible time of life. Life is just not worth living anymore. It's so humiliating to have to depend on others. I would just as soon pass on and get it over with." Please don't let this happen to you. I care very much that you have a happy future, and I'm here to cheer you on. So prepare for your future years. After all, one of the definitions of maturity is the willingness to forego some of today's pleasures for the sake of tomorrow's benefits. Except that today's pleasures need not be foregone. In fact the judicious and prudent preparation for your twilight years can be downright enjoyable, somewhat of a hobby, more enjoyable and profitable than raising fine roses. Get started now if you haven't done so. Don't miss the boat by standing on the pier too long.

One day when the trans-continental railroad was being laid, work was interrupted for a few minutes to honor Hop Sing, the proverbial Chinese cook.

A high-level superintendent said to his 200-or-so gathered workers, "We have an unsung hero among us. Hop Sing has been a huge asset to the company. For eight years he has consistently fed us enjoyable and nutritious meals every day without fail, and this kept the morale of all of us at a high level. He has never complained about anything. In appreciation of his long and faithful service I am happy to announce that we are raising Hop Sing's pay five-cents an hour. Do you agree that he deserves this raise?"

A mighty roar arose from the audience, a mixture of "Yes!" "Of Course!" "Sure!" "Yeah, Hop Sing!"

The superintendent beckoned Hop Sing to board the speakers' platform. When Hop Sing reluctantly did so, quiet suddenly settled on the crowd, because Hop Sing appeared to be sullen and unhappy, and perhaps even indignant.

The superintendent said, "Mr. Hop Sing, for your eight long years of faithful service to the company and your fellow employees, we are giving you a raise of five-cents-an-hour. Is there anything you would like to say at this time?"

Hop Sing slowly raised his head, looked his employer straight in the eye and said, "You clook me long time."

Don't you clook yourself long time.

Good health is your birthright. Don't give it up in exchange for a life of irresponsibility and superficial pleasures. True, we are put upon by hucksters from all sides, but it is not incumbent on us to help feather their nests. As Dr. Wayne Dyer says, no one can hurt you without your consent and cooperation. So if you would be healthy you must stop cooperating with those whose primary purpose in life is to separate you from your money. Take charge of yourself. Don't be satisfied with being anybody. Be somebody. I promise you, you'll find a pot of gold when you get there.

Remember this: You will be old. But you have been granted the privilege of determining whether you will be an "old man" or an "old woman," or whether you will be a healthy, lively well-seasoned person. When a doctor is stumped on your condition, he may ask, "How old are you?" Don't accept that kind of cop-out. It's not age that makes you old. It's you — and he.

I have chosen to categorize the requirements of health as follows: Cleanliness, Nutrition, Mind and Spirit, Exercise, and Rest. I'm designating Cleanliness the lead-off runner in order to give you a flying start in understanding my general theses on the requirements of health.

But before we get into our program, let me take a little time to first address the conscientious and exuberant among us:

If you're fed up with the status quo and are really committed to starting a new chapter on the state of your health, let me try to help you with a jet-assisted takeoff. Do the following things and you're well on your way to much better health:

+ Right now, if you're home, even if it's 2:00 a.m., take this book with you to your kitchen, and pull your large trash can out into the open.

+ Get your entire supply of sugar and dump it out, saying, "Out, you stupid thing!" If it's in a sack, open the sack and dump out the entire contents.

+ Do the same with all your white flour.

+ Dump everything that contains or is made of sugar and/or white flour, crumbling the cookies and obliterating the candy bars. Cuss at everything as you slam it into the trash.

+ Pour your sugared drinks down the drain. I'll allow you one last swig before you hang yourself. Don't fret; you will soon be born again.

+ Don't save your junk for Suzie or anyone else. Dump it. The more junk you have to "waste," the better. For results, quid pro quo works much better than free lunches.

+ If you're not home as you read this, do these things as soon as you get home, not after you change into your working clothes. Now. Pronto. If you have on a suit and tie, so much the better.

- Resolve not to buy or consume junk food in the future, including canned food.
- Resolve to buy and consume more fresh fruits, vegetables, seeds, nuts, and whole-grain cereals.
- Make good on these resolutions and continue to make good.

If somehow you are feeling a little better already, it's because you are a little healthier. I've told you that your mind and body are intimately interdependent.

We haven't brought up tobacco and alcohol yet. Let's do it now. If you now smoke and/or drink booze, dump those poisons too. Stomp or otherwise crush your last cigarettes. Empty your last bottle of booze.

Let me digress a bit and tell you of an experience related to what we've been discussing:

A few years ago my wife Janey and I had a business featuring body toning. A man of about forty came in purportedly to gather information for his wife about our health services. From across my desk he asked, "Mind if I smoke?" I said, "Yes," and pointed to a sign on the wall which said, "Thank you for not smoking." He said, "Good. I don't want to smoke anyway. Been trying to quit for years."

I asked, "How serious are you about wanting to quit?"

"Genuinely serious," he said.

"Okay. Let me see your cigarettes."

Larry handed me his cigarettes. By now I knew his name. I said, "With your permission I'd like to stomp on your cigarettes."

"That won't do any good. I've got six more packs at home."

"Go home and stomp on them too."

"Man, it's not my nature to waste like that. I'm not even working."

"It wouldn't be a waste. It would be a small investment to save you much more for the rest of your life, not to mention better health. Besides, you're wasting a lot now, especially since you're not working.

"Uh, uh. I'd give 'em to my friend."

I said, "If you're really serious about kicking the stupid weed listen to the pro and do as I say."

"What's wrong about giving the weed to a friend who has to buy the stuff every day? At least it won't be wasted."

"I told you it wouldn't be wasted. Okay, let me explain. When you stomp on your cigarettes you'll be paying a price for the freedom you've been trying to win. And that's good. You know there's no free lunch. When you pay for your freedom you'll duly appreciate it. Get it free and you'll take it cheap and probably smoke again."

Larry just smiled and looked at me. I tossed his cigarettes on the floor and stomped 'em real good, as we say in Tennessee. Then I reached into my cash drawer, pulled out two one-dollar bills, and handed them to Larry. He ignored them.

His smile broke out into more of a laugh. "Okay, okay. I'll go home and stomp the hell outa my six packs. He stood up and said, "Wish me luck!"

"You don't need any luck from me and you don't need wishbone. All you need is backbone."

As Larry went through the door he said, "Consider it done. Thanks!"

It wasn't long before I forgot all about Larry and his weed. But one day about six months later I went out to my car which was parked in front of our salon. There I noticed a lady walking toward me with a mile-wide smile on her face. She asked, "Are you the man who owns Slim City?" When I said I was she asked, "Do you remember the man

234

whom you advised to stomp on his cigarettes?" When I said yes again she said, "Well, he's my husband and he sent me to see you with a message. I didn't just drop in to see you. I came out of my way to deliver the message. Larry told me to tell you he's very grateful to you and that he hasn't smoked since."

I said, "Well, thanks for the happy message. Please tell Larry I'm happy for him."

Now you understand why I emphasize that you dump your junk instead of giving it to Suzie. If you do give it to anyone you will get gratitude in return and thus will not be paying a price for your freedom. So if you've got the gumption, go for it. But I'm not going to wish you luck, because wishing will not make it so. Backbone beats wishbone any time.

Easier said than done? Yes, but that's exactly what I did some forty years ago. The results I got were so dramatic that my excitement will remain with me the rest of my days. I'm so thankful for my body's ability to respond to my efforts that I feel obligated to my Creator to tell you that you can do the same.

But specifically what can you expect in return for all that enjoyable junk you sacrificed? Given that we're all at least a little different from one another, I can't make any solid specific promises, but I can say this with some confidence: If you do all the things I recommended above, you will be miles ahead on the road to health, provided, of course, you're not already pretty healthy. It is not an exaggeration to say that the moment you make the move, your body will make a U-turn and begin to prepare you for health. In a few weeks, or perhaps even days, you will actually feel the difference. If you have chronic symptoms, some of them may surprise you by fading away. But a few deep-seated symptoms, such as atherosclerosis, arthritis, and prostatitis may not be so easily eradicated. However, with some additional measures they too can be overcome, or at least alleviated. These additional measures may include fasting, chelation, a healthy state of mind, exercise, and judicious rest. These measures will be discussed soon.

Attention, please: After a few days of clean living you may experience a "cleansing reaction;" namely, bad feelings of some kind, or symptoms. If this happens to you, don't let it throw you, because this is a constructive, and beneficial event, the natural process of detoxification you've been working for. This is made possible by your having freed your body from their former task of keeping you from breaking down. Now that you have stopped piling in the garbage, your glands and other organs can now spend their time and energy shoveling the remaining garbage down the garbage chute. And if the purging is faster than your physiology can handle in a timely fashion by means of its usual, or normal, exits, Mother helps out by opening up additional exits; like perhaps a boil, a cold, a rash, more dandruff, sinuses, bad breath, a heavily coated tongue, and a variety of other symptoms. Even certain aches and pains, such as a headache or a fever, can result from the trauma of an excessively fast clean-up job. If this cleansing reaction is too discomforting for you, and since Socrates advised us to "Be moderate in all things," you have my permission to decrease the stringency of your dietary program in order to make your situation less stressful. But please do not completely abort your cleansing process. A caveat: You may feel so miserable that it may be difficult to believe you're getting healthy. But remember what we have been saying; that symptoms are a sign that your body is working to restore your health.

Stay on your winning horse. Increase and sustain your interest in health. See the other side of the mountain. Join a health club if you can find one. Or start one of your own. Subscribe to a good health magazine. "Prevention," an old standby, is a good one, but as far as I can judge, it has sold its soul to Big Medi$in. It has advertised drugs for several years. It has even sided with the Establishment in a vital controversy against the health people. The issue was political with potentially dire consequences. I'm almost certain it is now owned by one of our big pharmaceutical companies, probably Upjohn.

But fret not, because I will suggest to you an outfit you will like much better. It is the National Health Federation. (We discussed this organization in the chapter on Big Medi$in, but since not everybody reads a book in the usual manner, from front to back, a repetition here should be helpful to some.) The Federation is much better because in addition to grinding out an abundance of scientifically informative articles it participates aggressively in the perpetual fight for health freedom. Membership entitles you to its super monthly magazine the "Health Freedom News."

What health freedom is there to fight for? Plenty. Remember when it was a crime to use laetrile, even by the terminal cancer patient? Wasn't that an evil, tyrannical, dictatorial, high-handed law? You can thank the national Health Federation for having been a major factor in the hard-fought eradication of that inhumane law. For many years the Food and Drug Administration (your own FDA), staunchly supported by its partners in the Unholy Trinity, has been trying very hard to prohibit the sale of natural food supplements except by prescription from M.D.s. They try to accomplish this by declaring that natural food items carried in health food stores are drugs and therefore

237

dangerous and should be under the supervision of Medical Doctors, who know next to nothing about health and are really disease merchants. That fight is still ongoing, tooth and toenail. The NHF has been our stalwart champion in this frustrating and discouraging fight all these years. If you have kept up with this fiasco and if you knew the characters involved as I do, you would also feel that were it not for the perseverance of the Federation we would today be needing a medical prescription to buy sunflower seeds and safflower oil.

By becoming a member of the NHF you will participate in its noble endeavors for human rights. Aside from that, every month in the Health Freedom News you will receive a wealth of highly practical health information. The articles, though scientifically oriented, are thoroughly readable, digestible, and assimilable.

Let me excerpt from the magazine some of the things the Federation does. It:

♦ is working for your right to choose your own doctor, diet, and therapy.

♦ believes you have the right to take vitamins and nutritional supplements, and fights the drug company cronies in the FDA who want vitamins regulated as drugs.

♦ works for the passage of effective health freedom legislation at the local, state, and national levels.

♦ campaigns to kill bad legislation, such as forced fluoridation, when it denies you freedom to choose.

♦ upholds individual and family health rights through legal action.

♦ keeps its members abreast of legal, legislative, and scientific health controversies with special mailings and through its monthly magazine.

+ does what no other organization in the nation is doing to help Americans stay healthy and enjoy individual liberty.
+ is working for a better tomorrow today.
+ uses your annual dues to finance its continuing legislative, judicial, and educational drives for health freedom and happiness.

Regular membership annual dues are $36; seniors, $24; students, $24; foreign residents, $48.

Address of the NHF:

The National Health Federation
P.O. Box 688
Monrovia, CA 91016
Telephone (818) 357-2181

I personally regard membership in the NHF as one of the best things you as a health seeker can do for yourself and your family. I am confident you will find the magazine more enjoyable and beneficial that I could describe here.

Let's get on with our study.

VERY SPECIAL NOTES

Unless you are an atypical American in very good health with extraordinary knowledge of the true workings of your body (not what Big Medi$in teaches you), the probability is high that these special notes hold some benefit for you. They are special because their messages are not ones you hear every day; they are not included in the wisdom of Big Med. If one, two, or all three apply to you, their impact on your life and health can be considerable.

I don't have to tell you that millions of Americans are walking around in a quandary wondering why their health is always sub-par despite all the efforts to treat it right. They are frustrated by doctor after doctor who are doing nothing for them, but a lot to them. Some are told their problems are psychosomatic, or that they have a negativistic turn of mind or spirit. Some are finally compelled to conclude that they just come from fragile stock.

Here I will discuss only three of the causes of this general malaise. I believe them to be among the most common and least known.

INTESTINAL FLORA

It is sad enough that all people who adhere to the Standard American Diet (SAD) carry a portable cesspool around in their bodies. Still, Mother, forgiving as she is, tries her best to keep them functioning fairly well. These people may get along well enough, though they will die prematurely at 75 or 80 after a miserable "old age." But some are not so fortunate. Something is always wrong with their health, wrong enough to distinctly lower their quality of life. In these cases it is not only the SAD that is keeping its adherents always sick.

This unhappy condition often comes on abruptly, prevails the rest of the person's life, and its cause is never discovered. Most conventional doctors seem oblivious to this diseased state. So I will have to tell you. If you already know about this, good for you.

Here's what often happens. Let's say you're in pretty good shape but something small bothers you and you run to your doctor. He says. "Your temperature is up a bit, indicating that you have an infection of some kind. It appears minor but let's get it out of the way and get you feeling comfortable. Here's the prescription. Follow the instructions and you'll be okay soon."

Well, Doc was right — somewhat. The infection is gone and you feel better. Except that now you're constipated. You probably don't correlate your constipation with your antibiotic treatment. But not to worry. You just take care of it with a laxative, which relieves the difficulty. However, the constipation returns in a few days, followed by diarrhea. You seem to be producing a lot of gas too. Well this should go away in time. Nothing is forever. But it doesn't go away and in fact gets worse. You just don't feel right. Your morale and disposition suffer, and eventually you go to the doctor again, and he prescribes another round of antibiotics. "This should take care of it." But it doesn't, and eventually you go back to him. He says, "We're all built differently. You seem to be more prone to digestive and eliminative disorders. The smart thing to do is to accept them and take a good laxative when you need it. Free your mind for more important things." You are frustrated with Doc's defeatist attitude but what can you do but go along with it?

You may not realize it but the antibiotics are what did it to you. They are not selective in whom they kill. So your acidophilus bacteria, your God-given beneficial ones which keep your digestion and elimination running right, are killed along with the harmful ones. And so, after your regimen of antibiotics, your intestines are practically devoid of bacteria of any kind, and now it's a toss-up as to which organism will thrive and occupy your gut. Now, if you observe a good, clean diet, your benevolent acidophilus will gradually build up and prevail, restoring a healthy condition to your system. But if you persist in consuming the SAD, the undesirable bugs, now free of competition for space, will take over and keep you in an unhealthy state, possibly for the rest of your life if you don't wise up and stop feeding these cesspool-type bacteria. Incidentally, the cesspool bugs we're talking about are predominantly Escherichia coli, which we're hearing more about recently and which have become more aggressive and murderous of late, having been challenged by antibiotics to protect themselves by producing more powerful and resistant strains of themselves. When I studied bacteriology in 1937, E.Coli was not the scary monster it is now.

Now, hold it! Let's not go bad-mouthing the E.coli. They don't wear black hats. Their God-given function is to process and get rid of trash, returning it to the dust from whence we came. So if you keep feeding them trash, what should you expect? Who's to blame, really? On the other hand, the acidophilus have the responsibility of converting the real food into healthy blood and tissues. This is the good ol' division of labor principle at work. Too simplistic? Too cut and dried? But that is how it is. It helps to remember that God did not surround us with enemies.

Remember also that to a great degree death begins in the colon. So if you care about your health, if you appreciate Mother's Marvelous Machine, help her take care of you. Do you part, then get out of her way. You do this by eating only food in as natural a state as possible, unblemished by the hand of man. Observe a few other rules of health and you've got it made. You'll find some of the rules soon.

DENTAL FILLINGS

This subject is raging controversy and I'm tempted to ask why it should be so controversial when the facts are so obvious — to me at least. "Amalgam" is used by mainstream dentists to fill cavities in teeth and accepted by the industry as being non-toxic and harmless. On the other hand, many people including some dentists vehemently maintain that the mercury in the amalgam is responsible for much human misery. The composition of the amalgam differs, though not significantly, between dentists, but typically it contains 50 percent mercury and the remainder comprises silver, zinc, and copper. Mercury is highly toxic and described by some as one of the most toxic chemicals known to man. It is used in the amalgam to provide pliability and workability, thus facilitating the task of packing it into the tooth cavity. The other components are there to provide body, because when the mercury eventually dissipates the filling will still be there, though reportedly many fillings have fallen out when enough mercury has "gassed out."

Several decades ago, some members of the American Dental Association (ADA) stepped forward and said, "Hey, fellas, we think we're doing something terribly wrong for our patients. It appears the mercury in our amalgam fillings are poisoning them. Some of it seems to be leaching out and getting into the systems of the patients, some of whom are getting very sick from it."

"Bah, humbug! No such thing. How can the mercury escape when it is all bound up in a compound of several metals?"

"What do you mean, 'no such thing'? There certainly is such a thing. The mercury is not bound up in a compound. It is a mixture, not a compound. It is impossible to create a compound of four metals."

The metals are still pure metals, mixed with one another. There is no such thing as mercuric silver. Metals simply do not react together to form compounds. So the leaching of the metals is only inhibited, or slowed, from leaving the group only by the close physical proximity of the components. Given the extreme toxicity of mercury and the amount of time available for it to do its thing, it works subtly and sometimes not so subtly to keep the patient in poor health, usually for the rest of his life. The fillings are called "silver" apparently because they then sound more innocent than "mercury" fillings.

Very sophisticated instruments have been designed and produced to measure the amount of mercury gases escaping from the fillings.

One dentist tried to pull the "compound" theory on me. "The mercury cannot escape the fillings, because it's held in place by the other components of the compound." I thought, "You've been through dental school and should know better. Either you're stupid or think I'm stupid enough to buy that stuff." Another dentist was more honest. He didn't answer my question, merely gave me a few copies of the ADA's propaganda.

The dissension in the ADA eventually caused a breakup of the group, and the main body of the Association is still alive and well, as is the wholesale use of the mercury fillings. Is conventional wisdom always right? Does the truth always prevail? You know my opinion. The anti-mercury camp seems to make more sense. What do you think?

CAUTION: If you buy my anti-mercury rationale, it's only logical that you should ask your dentist to replace your "silver fillings" with some non-toxic material. But it's not that simple. According to specialists in the field, the sequence of the amalgam removals can be critical; an incorrect sequence can bring you big-time health problems. If you wan to speak with experts in this field of dentistry, I suggest you contact the following:

Higgins Diagnostic Center
5080 List Drive, at Centennial
Colorado Springs, CO 80919
Telephone (719) 548-1600

Higgins seems to be the foremost pioneer in this very specialized discipline. You may travel to Colorado Springs to consult with them and have them do your dental work, or you might telephone them to ask them to refer you to a specialist near you whom they approve of for performing that type of esoteric work.

But do you remember what I told you about alternative physicians' being as human as the mainstream physicians and possessing the same appreciation of the finer things of life? Well, remember also that alternative dentists are human too and also share the love of the finer things. Whether their beneficial services are worth what they charge you is not for me to say. But I will submit, for whatever my judgment is worth, that a healthy dental condition is a very valuable asset which will enhance your whole being.

DENTAL ROOT CANALS

The patient has a toothache and goes to see his dentist, who takes an x-ray shot and concludes that the decay is pretty deep. "Sorry, Robert, but filling won't solve your problem. We have to either pull the tooth or root-canal it. I presume you prefer to have it canaled.

"You can say that again. Anything to save my tooth is better than losing it and having to wear some clumsy contraption in my mouth."

So Dr. Yankum gets out his drill and long fluted cleaner-outer and draws out the pulp from the sick tooth. And now everything is okay again. Robert has a dead tooth but it does the job and won't be subject to decay anymore.

But wait a minute. That's not necessarily true. I won't pretend to know everything about the effects of root canaling and so I will leave this question up to you. I can only tell you what I have been told by supposedly sophisticated health-oriented dentists and let you decide the facts for yourself. So here is the explanation:

A tooth is made up of three parts: the dentine, which is the main body of the tooth; the protective enamel on the outside; and the pulp, the soft core of the tooth. Some teeth don't have simple, straight roots and pulps; and so some of the pulp cannot be drawn out and must remain in the tooth to support further decay. But let's talk about a tooth with a straight root and pulp. Is the tooth now safe from further decay? No, not at all, according to the specialists. The dentine is organic material and is now dead too. Remember that germs have the job of processing dead organic materials and returning them to dust to keep the wonderful life cycle intact. So the dentine, somewhat softer than the enamel, is now food for the microbes, who duly go to work to fulfill their purpose. Because the nerve has been removed from the tooth Robert now feels no pain and is oblivious to the feast now going on in his mouth. But the feast gives rise to a low-grade infection, pain or no pain, which, albeit subtle, jeopardizes Robert's health to at least a significant degree.

If you're reading this, you're obviously not only six years old. And the chances are pretty good that you're carrying around a few root canals yourself. So what can you do to protect your health form the toxic effects of your dental condition? (1) You can disregard this theory as just so much propaganda, (2) You can accept this subtle infection and quit worrying about it, (3) You can ask Dr. Yankum to extract the tooth and replace it with some clumsy contraption, or (4) You can do none of the above, since they all are unsatisfactory at best. Here's my favorite approach to dental health; regardless of whatever else I do: Keep my whole body healthy and invulnerable to any adverse influences. It's really not very difficult once you accept the responsibility of being a good steward of your wonderful body. We will discuss the requisites for health in the following pages.

I realize that the details of health concerns can be nettling in a life already overburdened with details. But you must decide one way or the other, because to not decide to care is to decide not to care. How important is health to you? It's up to you. Your health is very important to me.

INNER CLEANLINESS

The word "clean" or "cleanliness," for our purposes here and unless otherwise expressed, will denote internal cleanliness. External cleanliness, aside from social considerations, pales into comparative insignificance. Further, be it known that I unequivocally reject the germ theory. We have already discussed our microscopic friends. When I speak of cleanliness I will not be referring to sanitation and the ramifications that word traditionally connotes. The adverse factors which give rise to internal uncleanliness are more often toxins and free radicals.

Obviously no one requisite alone when satisfied will result in good health, but if I were compelled to name the most important requirement, I would be hard-pressed to choose between cleanliness and good nutrition, because these two

247

are so interdependent, more so than love and marriage, that you can't have one without the other. But fortunately we don't have to choose. No matter what other beneficial things you do for your body, it simply will not thrive when the cells of all its parts are impregnated with sludge and unable to utilize the materials required to build it into the sturdy and efficient machine which is necessary for an optimally successful life. Good food is largely wasted in a congested body. If that is not enough to justify top billing for cleanliness consider that toxemia, a poisoned condition of the body, is a primary requirement for atherosclerosis, arthritis, cancer, and other chronic symptoms of disease.

The toxins which debilitate your health come from outside and inside your body. The outside ones invade your body by way of your mouth, lungs, and skin. The inside ones develop in the course of the body's metabolism.

Use of the word "natural" has proliferated and crescendoed on our supermarket shelves, demonstrating that even mainstream industry has jumped on the health bandwagon, finding a seat next to those who were once known derisively as "health nuts." Clearly the consumer increasingly appreciates that natural is better than adulterated and fragmented. Only recently has Big Medi$in jumped on, but it is still milking its own propaganda on health and disease for whatever value it has left, before it finally and belatedly decides to find a permanent seat and preach to the consumer what it will try to pass off as its very own advice and recommendations. "If you can't lick 'em, join 'em." Thus it has ever been.

Though probably a good majority of us now somehow sense that natural food is better for us, our knowledge of why this is so is at best nebulous and not quite definitive enough to inspire us to pursue health in earnest. So let me try to add to your perspective in hopes that you will thus become a somewhat better steward of your God-given body.

Why the big to-do over "natural"? First and obviously, before the advent of the industrial revolution not very much more than a century ago, man lived with nature for eons on end. A hundred-and-fifty years is an extremely short interval in the evolution of man, not nearly enough time to adjust to drastically new environmental conditions. Neither can he cope with foods stripped of their beneficial factors and left incomplete and thus incapable of participating in the intended organic reactions which would otherwise render them part of the body. Left out of the action, the erstwhile "food" is now excess baggage, more accurately, garbage. Together with the extraneous chemicals alluded to above, it is now poison. It is intentionally that I paint that word poison with a broad brush, because it is just that, poison. Anything that is not metabolic material, used as a building block for the body, is not only extraneous and useless, but also very damaging as it stands in the way of body functions.

In eons past, this poisonous material was not much of a problem, because then man ate only natural foods, and not an overabundance of them either. And what little useless food factors remained unassimilated after processing was easily purged by way of natural physiological functions. But today, with the unnatural quantities of industrial chemicals poured through his gullet, lungs, and skin, as well as the food factors isolated by food processors and thus converted to garbage, man simply cannot keep up in his body's attempt to free itself of the garbage. The backlog becomes sludge and eventually impregnates every cell in the body.

"If the situation is as bad as you make it out to be, how come I don't see everybody getting sick?" Are you kidding? Then why is it that we Americans spend such a huge proportion of our income to hire doctors to abort our symptoms, effectively blocking off our garbage chutes, only to have Mother try other avenues of escape which may in turn also be blocked off? Etcetera, etcetera, etcetera? And why are we dying prematurely after only eighty years of a sick life?

Big Med has made an efficient science of eliminating the pain of symptoms, thus not only aborting the cleansing process but also intercepting Mother's message, "My child, better get on the ball. Your body needs your attention." Good doctors, whose side are you on?

I promised you I would harp on, and repeat, one of the major theses on which this book is built, and this is as good a time as any to do it: There is only one disease, a generally deteriorated body. What are popularly called diseases are but local expressions of the one disease, avenues by which the body attempts to purge itself. Any abortion of the process is a violation and frustration of nature and serves only to exacerbate the disease.

In the realm of physiological cleanliness the big negative concern is the free radical, which was discussed earlier. Free radicals are a wild and unruly entity which attacks our cells and debilitates our bodies, aging us prematurely. They are not really individual critters but more accurately and practically described as a polluted, or contaminated, state of our blood and tissues, including our vital organs. Though we can name numerous factors inimical to health, they all give rise to the free radical, which ultimately is the culprit who raises havoc by attacking our cells and embroiling our bodies into a diseased state.

Free radicals are a normal participant in a healthy person and are of little concern there, as the healthy body routinely renders them harmless. But in our modern ways of life free radicals are imposed on our systems in such excessive quantities that we are hard-pressed to tolerate them without incurring some degree of chronic illness.

But the effects of free radicals would be much worse, in fact intolerable, were it not for a mitigating factor known as antioxidants, so named because they prevent oxidation, which in this context means putrefaction and contamination, or toxemia. You will recall that a free radical is an oxygen molecule with an unpaired electron in search of a partner and as such is very reactive and disruptive of normal body conditions. The antioxidant protects us by inhibiting the feisty radical in its mischievous work. Like free radicals, antioxidants occur naturally in our bodies, but not in sufficient quantities to adequately negate the effects of abnormally large quantities of free radicals. And so health-conscious persons try to decrease their quantities of free radicals by consuming more natural, real foods and shunning junk. They also increase their supply of antioxidants in the form of food supplements, a few of which are vitamin C, vitamin E, beta carotene, and selenium.

For years, indeed decades, vitamins C and E have been described as being very good for our health but not much was said about what they do for us, except that they helped prevent, and also combatted, infection. Now that they are called antioxidants, or free radical scavengers, we should have a better handle on these two health aids and know better how to regard and use them.

In recent years another antioxidant, named pycnogenol, has become immensely popular. It is purported to be 20 times as effective as vitamin C and 50 times as effective as

251

vitamin E in scavenging free radicals. After personally using pycnogenol and experiencing its results I am thoroughly sold on it. Interestingly, it is not a new discovery. It's been known for several centuries but only a few years ago became duly appreciated for its capabilities. People in other countries have used it for several years now, especially in Europe and Japan. Though it has been slow making its mark in America, its virtues have made its eventual popularity inevitable. So highly regarded is it that it is now the object of many multi-level sales programs across the continent. But don't ask your MD about pycnogenol. As a health enhancer it is not in his world.

Incidentally, the two major sources from which pycnogenol is extracted are (1) the bark of the marine pine tree, which grows extensively in southern Europe and (2) grape seeds, consequently now a significant by-product of the wine industry. It seems likely that new sources will be scouted for, discovered, and exploited, with favorable effects on cost and pricing.

By the time you read this you very probably will have heard of another extremely popular elixir: kombucha, also known as mushroom tea, Manchurian tea, champignon de longue vie, and a list of names too long and impractical to mention. It has found its way over the breadth of our nation and very possibly across the entire continent. Its virtues are legendary, and my very firm opinion, along with those of many of its other users, is that it's a Real McCoy and not a mere fad. The wild stories told about its results appear to be well founded.

Like pycnogenol, it was slow making it to the U.S. But unlike pycnogenol, it has been used as a health tonic since well before the time of Christ. It apparently originated in China and eventually spread to other Asiatic countries including Russia, then to India, Spain, and other European countries.

It would serve no practical purpose to try to tell you everything about this endearing mushroom, but I'll say this: Get it if you can. And I'm fairly sure it's widespread enough that you will be able to find one. But don't buy it. One of the big rules about kombucha is that it should not be sold, but given away free and with love. Though botanically it is a fungus, or mushroom, it looks like a flat gelatinous pancake and reproduces a "baby" mushroom every few days. The baby is kept and the "mama" is given away. And on and on it goes, spreading health benefits among your family and other loved ones. It is customary that the giver also give to the giftee a copy of the instructions on the history and use of kombucha. So I'll leave you in the hands of the person who loves you enough to give you kombucha.

We have asked why "natural," and perhaps have increased our perspective enough to ask what is natural. Natural food is whole food as it comes from nature, no more and no less; nothing artificial added and none of its essentials taken away. Some of the supplements we swallow are whole foods and some are not. For example, desiccated liver is, or is supposed to be, merely whole healthy calves' liver dried and marketed as tablets for convenience. It is valued because it is known to be very rich in the B vitamins and certain other beneficial nutriments. In the drying process high temperatures are avoided in order to preserve the delicate and elusive enzymes and other factors which are destroyed by heat. Pure vitamin C is pure ascorbic acid, which can be, and sometimes is, extracted from non-food sources. True, it is comparatively inexpensive and does provide significant benefits, but it is not a whole food and in fact not a food at all. It lacks the accompanying ingredients which in nature do their work synergistically in concert with the vitamin C and one another.

So why natural foods? Again, for eons man lived with and adapted to natural foods. Even without today's high-tech, he managed to unwittingly get his share of the vitamins A, B, C, D, E, F, G, and K, the bioflavonoids, the minerals, antioxidants, chlorophyll, digestive aids, enzymes, omega-3 fatty acids, acidophilus, fiber, fructose, and all the wonderful health factors we try so hard to obtain today, some of which are attainable only with the help of high-tech laboratory research; as well as, undoubtedly, many beneficial health factors as yet still unknown to man.

Just a few decades ago someone discovered vitamin B-12, and the whole world exclaimed, "We've got a miracle vitamin!" Even the medical industry uncharacteristically jumped on the wagon, obviously because the benefits of B-12 were so substantial that they couldn't be naysayed without sounding stupid, and perhaps also because the vitamin could be administered through their profitable needles. But you know what? The health nuts who had been taking brewer's yeast and desiccated liver, as well as fresh liver, were getting vitamin B-12 into their bodies all along. That's just one example of why natural foods. The same concept applies ad infinitum concerning other nutriments and the "natural" foods containing them.

What starts out as God-given food soon starts on its journey to become unnatural. Some seeds are chemicalized. The plants are fed products of the chemistry laboratory and then sprayed with other chemicals which are absorbed by the foliage and thus carried into our bodies. Livestock is raised under stressful and unnatural conditions and injected with drugs to induce unnatural growth. Our manufactured chicken eggs are a far cry from what our grandparents ate.

The food processors and packers get hold of our food and really do a job on it. They add to it, subtract from it, divide it, and multiply the woes of the consumer. The chemicals are added in such quantities that the average American now consumes about eight pounds of it per year, not including sugar. That's several teaspoonsful of a complement of various high-tech chemicals per day! They also fragment many foods and discard some of the parts, leaving the remainder stranded as garbage and consumed supposedly as food.

Now, it is not my intent to derogate the farmers and food processors. They are in business to give the consumer what he wants at the price he wants to pay for it. What else can they do and yet stay in business? You the consumer in effect are the party calling the shots, and this is a big reason a book like this should be addressed to the consumer. You are in position to demonstrate to the marketers what foods you want to buy and how you want them prepared and marketed.

The same concept applies to your relationship with your doctors. Officially they are not motivated by altruism. I can't blame them either for what they are doing to us, even if I dislike their medical concepts. As long as you roll up your sleeve or pull down your pants for them, they will stick it to you. As long as you're happy to give the pharmacist your money, the good doctor will continue to tell you what drug you need today. As long as you sign the papers, he's willing to wield the scalpel. Remember, to the man with a hammer in his hand everything looks like a nail. So as long as you provide the demand, someone will gladly provide the supply and gladly take your money. Ultimately you call the shots.

Let me give you a real, everyday example of how our food is ruined in deference to profit — and, of course, you the consumer want it that way. The wheat grain is an ingeniously packaged do-it-yourself nourishment kit. It is dried to prevent premature blending of its three parts: a starchy body called the endosperm; the germ, a storehouse of nutriments; and the bran, a protective wrapping which also serves a function in the digestive and eliminative processes. When the grain is chewed and moistened with saliva, the three parts combine and together serve the purpose of nourishing the body. They would nourish the body, that is, if we let them do it. But we don't let them, because the general practice in the "civilized" world is to separate the three parts and use only the starchy endosperm as human food. It is now known as white flour.

So what is wrong with white flour? Well, when Mr. Starchy Endosperm gets into your insides and ready to work, he'll find himself all alone without his teammates and unable to convert into blood and tissue. Without the other ingredients all he can do is to provide temporary energy. So far, not too bad. But what becomes of him? Some of him is stored as fat. Since he cannot become part of you, he's not only useless, for the most part, but he's also garbage. Trouble is, he probably can't be shipped out yet, if ever, because there's a long line of garbage ahead of him waiting its turn at the chute. And there we have those old free radicals again. Considering all the white flour and other goofed-up foods we consume, including more than a half-cup of sugar daily, is it any wonder we're so sick? Is it any wonder that cancer is now the leading killer of children? Isn't it a wonder we aren't even sicker than we are?

Refined flour and sugar aren't the only tempting man-made pseudo-foods that are landing us in the hospital more than necessary and underground before our time. Very few foods escape man's folly. And happily the few that do are increasingly consumed by a growing number of enlightened persons who value their health and realize that the food and medical industries are not obsessed with a concern for the welfare of their customers. These persons have determined that the Little Red Hen was right all along.

"Hey, you said that life is to be enjoyed, that we should not go overboard on this health thing. At least white flour and sugar aren't carcinogens, and that's a good compromise." Yes, life is to be enjoyed, and I want very much for you to enjoy it. But which part of it do you want to enjoy? It depends a lot on what you call enjoyment. If you habitually consume the Standard American Diet (the SAD), it is doubtful that you will be able to fully enjoy both ends of your life. Look around you at our seniors and think it over for yourself.

But who says white flour and white sugar aren't carcinogens? A carcinogen in my book (pun not intended) is anything that tends to eventually give rise to the development of cancer or leads in the direction of cancer. Since cancer is the ultimate failure of the body, anything that undermines your health leads in the direction of cancer. Don't let those erudite men of the medical and pharmaceutical industries hoodwink you into standing in awe of their unwarrantedly complicated theories on cancer. They may be correct, which I have come to doubt, but all of their moot information is valued only because we have wantonly refused to live responsibly. I'm not an oncologist and neither are you, so all we care about are the practical facts as they apply to our not being the one-in-three Americans who will some day be struck down by cancer. Look at the facts as you believe them to be and then decide for yourself how much you want to, or don't want to, compromise with your non-carcinogens.

Please understand, I'm not pitting my hypoglycemic brain against the genius of the MDs and PhDs. I learned my facts from the late Max Gerson, who was described by no less than Dr. Albert Schweitzer as "the greatest genius in the history of medicine." But I didn't take even Dr. Schweitzer's word for it; I thoroughly studied Dr. Gerson myself. Study him yourself and your perspective can only be enhanced for it. If you don't know of Max Gerson, it is probably because he was heavily persecuted by Big Medi$in with the solid help of the U.S. Congress. His crime was curing cancer too consistently. He was bullied out of New York, then out of New Jersey. The Gerson Institute is now in California and does not have a hospital but works together with a Mexican hospital in Tijuana. This seems to be the only arrangement which will keep Big Medi$in off his back. The Institute is now operated by the late Dr. Gerson's daughter, Charlotte Gerson. Its mailing address is P.O. Box 430; Bonita, CA 91908. The telephone number is (619) 267-1150.

Dr. Gerson said that cancer results when the body fails to produce an "allergic inflammation." First you should know that an allergic inflammation, like other symptoms we experience, is a beneficial reaction, a protective, defensive, normalizing one. So when a body becomes so degenerated that it no longer can protect itself, cancer occurs. In plain words, cancer is the ultimate state of the one disease. The progression of any illness leads in the direction of cancer.

What is this protection that we allude to that the body normally affords itself? It is the beneficent work of the glands and other organs, as well as all the rest of the physiology. When the body becomes impregnated by extraneous materials, the organs work hard at normalizing the conditions, purging the impurities. But remember, the organs are an integral part of the body and are susceptible also to the disabling effects of the toxins. So when the body becomes so degenerated that even the benevolent organs are incapacitated, that's cancer. And since only the body, with Mother's help, can cure itself, the only thing man can do to rid himself of cancer is to purge the entire body of impurities and provide nourishment to rebuild the tissues while restoring the normal capabilities of the organs, which will then resume their normal duties and try to restore health. These, in brief, are the measures undertaken by the Gerson clinic, and this is how they cure so many, even terminal cases. One must wonder why our MDs think they can cut, poison, and burn their patients to health.

Consume enough charred fats, rancid food, salt, chemically cured meats, chemical food additives, white flour and sugar, and you can be a victim of cancer. Likewise if you breathe too many aromatic fumes or coal dust, or soak your hands in too many strong chemicals, or sustain too many and too severe emotional stresses. In short, all influences inimical to health are carcinogens.

You know, of course, that it is not my intent that you live in fear of all the bad things just mentioned above. I went to the extreme in order to point out the direction of cancer, so to speak. It is for you to decide how far you are willing to go in that direction.

Let's push the concept of free radicals a little further. Any influence that destroys the natural state of food produces free radicals and is inimical to health, and of course, strictly speaking, carcinogenic. Even ordinary cooking is harmful; overcooking is worse. When enzymes and other food factors are destroyed, their intended transformation into blood and tissue is short-stopped, and the factors remaining are no longer food but will be garbage if taken into the body. This is why we have so many raw-food advocates among the serious health seekers these days.

Let's talk a little of how toxins and free radicals are created in the body. Stresses are the common denominator in the processes. Physical trauma (accidental injuries) produces toxins, because tissues are destroyed and thus transformed into dead matter, and we know that dead matter is garbage. Emotional trauma is not merely an ethereal will o' the wisp with no physical connections. We have already said that the body, including the brain, is an integration of all its parts working interdependently in harmony with one another. The mind is a product of the brain, and there can be no thought without the brain. Much physical energy is required to run the brain, and conversely emotional and mental trauma weigh heavily on the brain, the other nerves, and the entire body. Incidentally, the brain is just one big nerve, and the nervous system is actually an electrical system. Thoughts and emotions are electrical impulses. In view of all this we can understand that good physical health is extremely important, in fact essential, to good mental health. I should know, because, as I have related earlier, hypoglycemia utterly ruined my scholastic career, as well as other aspects of my life. I can easily understand why so many children, malnourished as many of them are these days, escape life by way of suicide. Hypoglycemia is implicated in alcoholism and other mental illnesses. But don't stand on your head while waiting for your friendly doctor to tell you this. In fact I would hold him in low esteem as a businessman if he did tell you this. But let me say this to you: If you are alcoholic or addicted in other ways, if you're allergic, if you suspect yourself of being a bit fuzzy-headed, look to physical health for a possible solution, especially your blood sugar health. I dare say that if the whole world were in good physical health, we would have much fewer radicals and terrorists and much more peace. J. Edgar Hoover, former chief of the FBI, also felt that faulty body chemistry was at the root of much crime and violence.

Physical exercise, in work or play, produces toxins. But in moderation that's okay, just normal routine. But when it is excessive, and excessive toxins are produced, the results could be detrimental.

Now comes a topic of perhaps greater importance: digestion, indigestion, and elimination. Jonn Matsen, N.D., of North Vancouver, B.C., makes a convincing case for indigestion's being a very major cause of disease. He does make sense when one considers the great quantities of material that are poured into the digestive system throughout the day, every day. On the basis that we are what we eat, apologies to the medical establishment, we can easily agree that what happens in our bodies in response to what we eat is of significant importance. Dr. Matsen's book, "Mysterious Cause of Illness," could be profitable reading.

Part of the digestive process occurs in the intestines. I place considerable emphasis on the importance of what happens here and so should you. In view of its direct influence on your health, it receives disproportionately little attention from Big Med — which is close to zero. So don't bother to ask your establishment doctor about it. He probably doesn't know about it and cares less. Except, of course, when an opportunity arises to put a scalpel to it.

All of us have numerous species and strains of bacteria in our intestines, some friendly and some unfriendly. Ideally, the predominant one should be Lactobacillus acidophilus and its relatives. But when junk food is consumed, and that is often, it increases the population of such as the unfriendly Escherichia coli, commonly known as E. coli. Yes, this is the same organism which was so heavily involved in the deaths of several children in the fast food restaurant episode not many years ago. It is also known as the cesspool bacterium and fosters an unhealthy condition of the bowels, including gas, constipation, diarrhea, diverticulosis, appendicitis, and regretfully colorectal cancer. But that's not all of it, not nearly all. An unhealthy intestinal flora is a major cause of general toxemia throughout the body. So much so that it has often been said by many health specialists that "Death begins in the colon." When I say that your establishment doctor knows very little about this, I am not being derogatory. I don't know whether this ignorance is by design, but unhealthy intestinal systems generate humongous volumes of business for them. It will behoove you to realize this as you navigate your way through the halls of medicine.

Because the intestinal flora is not one of the interests of Big Med, numerous people are walking around with lifetime indigestion, constipation, hemorrhoids, gas, and many seemingly unrelated miseries resulting therefrom. When antibiotics are administered to a patient, they are not very selective in whom they kill. If the dosage is strong enough, all or nearly all the bacteria die, our friendly acidophilus included. Now, if our medicated patient should consume only good food after his treatment, his friendly bacteria could thrive again and restore intestinal health. But given our junk food culture, most of us will continue to feed the cesspool organisms and thereby perpetuate intestinal pollution with its concomitant conditions of disease, which, as we have said, is a generally degenerated body.

So after antibiotic treatment we should be especially careful to maximize our consumption of clean foods; that is, foods in their most natural state possible, and minimize consumption of junk. If in spite of your efforts you still feel your gut health is not quite right, you might do well to reseed your system with acidophilus from the health food store and ingest a significant amount of live-culture yogurt for at least a while.

Refined sugar, both white and brown, and white flour are extremely detrimental to health. Sugar is by far the worse of the two, but the effects of white flour are generally similar to those of sugar. So we will confine our discussion to sugar and deduce our opinion of flour by extrapolation. To simplify, refined sugar will be expressed simply as sugar.

Simply put, sugar is simply horrible. It seems to contribute to almost all illnesses we experience. It engenders huge quantities of free radicals which result in our terrifying rates of heart disease, cancer, insanity, arthritis, and a seemingly endless list of other maladies. It so affects our metabolism that our aging clock runs at abnormal speed. The precocious sexual maturity of our children exemplifies this abnormal acceleration of aging. Notice the sexy appearance and demeanor of our teenagers and even some pre-teenagers.

Chronic disease runs rampant despite a significant increase in health knowledge. It is only people's obsession with appearance by way of high-tech cosmetics and sporty clothes that belies their true age and physical condition.

Is it mere coincidence that suicide is the leading killer of our young people and that they are also the ones who have grown up with junk food and don't know better?

Refined sugar is poison. Because it is not nearly a complete food it is in effect one big free radical, unfettered and free to wreak havoc with our cells and debilitate our bodies. It has enough despicable attributes to fill volumes, so I could not do the subject justice to try to paint a complete picture of it here. But it bears so heavily on your health that I strongly recommend that you go to your library and read some of the many books on the subject. A good one is "Sweet and Dangerous," by John Yudkin, M.D. You will find more recommended books in the Appendix.

Sugar and white flour are not by any means the only troublemakers in our bodies, merely among the worst. Their effects are more damaging than most partly because they are so popular and consumed in much greater quantities. As has been said earlier but worth repeating, all foods that are not whole foods, that have been contaminated with additives, including preservatives, that have lost some of their factors either by the hand of man or by staleness, have lost their wholesomeness and in varying degrees are toxic.

The detrimental effects of tobacco, alcohol, coffee, tea, and other drugs are so well known, having been drummed into us since kindergarten days, that to discuss them would be beating a dead horse. However, be informed that each little cigarette you smoke will take several minutes off your life span, while in the meantime taking quality off your life and health.

We have said that contaminants enter our bodies also through our lungs and our skin, but you can say that again, because this fact is given far too little consideration. While some of the absorption is almost inevitable, some of it is under our control. It may be unreasonable to expect you to avoid the smog of big cities, but you can easily minimize the inhalation of carcinogenic fumes at home. If you must spray your hair you don't have to stand or sit there and breathe in the surrounding mist of strong chemicals. And what about those 32 jars of mysterious potions that cover your dressing table? They are a veritable chemical laboratory: shampoo, conditioners, special rinses, hair dyes, curl holders, antiperspirants, deodorants, depilatories, perfume, colognes, after-shave, face and body lotions, nail polish, nail polish remover, astringent, cleansing creme, powder, rouge, mascara, eyebrow pencil, eye liner, eyelash thickener, shaving cream, mouth wash, toothpaste, eye drops, lipsticks, the pink stuff that coats, nasal spray, antihistamines, cough medicines, dandruff eliminators,... "Hey, hey, what are you trying to do, take away all my pleasures?" No, I'm just reminding you of all the unnatural chemicals you're inflating your lungs with and pushing through your skin and into your bloodstream. Behold the free radicals! Somewhere in those 32 containers there must be a few so-called carcinogens, although I feel they are all carcinogens and cumulatively could be deadly and probably are deadly. You deserve a fair chance to know what you're doing as you make your choices in managing your risks. We know that the incidence of breast cancer is already high and getting worse. Is it not reasonable to at least suspect a connection between breast cancer and vanity chemicals? We, all of us, are prone to turn the other way and ignore the risks in deference to creature comforts and pleasures. But perhaps it's a good idea to now and then turn our heads back straight and face our situation squarely, then make our choices. Your choice is your responsibility. My responsibility in writing this book is to try to enhance your life and happiness.

Notice that we have the means to stop the scalp from shedding dead skin, the sinuses from releasing their yuck, and perspiration from escaping the body, now all we need is a couple of stout plugs to finish the job.

The bathroom is not the only battlefield. The rest of the house is also a mine field. Oh, the delicious smell of our new carpet. And the draperies smell good too, fresh from the cleaners. And those air fresheners pasted up on the walls. And those little bowls of wood shavings impregnated with aromatic fragrances.

Some kitchen cabinets are not so obvious in their emission of toxic fumes. They are the ones made of certain kinds of particle board. The resin which holds the particles together contains formaldehyde, a seriously toxic substance, which is emitted into the house not only when new but for a long time following. This used to be a common condition, but I hope its inherent hazard has convinced the manufacturers to stop producing this type of material. Nevertheless, it would be very advisable before moving into a house or apartment to ascertain that the cabinets are formaldehyde-free.

Wall paint is another danger. The new types do not give off as much odor as the older types did, but they do emit their share of toxins.

And, oh, that delectable smell of a new car. Sorry, but that's full of carcinogens too.

And those efficient cleaning solvents we use around the house and in the garage; they're not innocent either. They penetrate your skin and mucus membranes as easily as they dissolve stubborn stains.

Every major brand of toothpaste in the U.S. contains sodium lauryl sulfate (Texapon), a foaming chemical which attacks the tissues of your mouth. This was announced by Klaus Bednarz in Hamburg, Germany. Did you expect to hear this from an American? But there's a serious risk only if the percentage of the stuff is more than two percent of the toothpaste. How much our toothpastes contain I don't know. So if you don't mind just a little poison twice a day, every day, I guess you can continue absorbing the stuff, even though 90 percent of it remains with you after rinsing and gargling. As for me, I suspected and quit using mainstream toothpaste three or four decades ago. Many shampoos also contain this chemical. Old Stick-in-the-Mud doesn't use shampoos either.

In October, 1992, a Los Angeles doctor transplanted a pig's liver into a woman. The reason given was a shortage of good human livers, which reportedly are increasingly difficult to obtain. Perhaps this demonstrates to us how our ways of living are affecting all of humanity.

I hope you are now more convinced than ever of the dangers inherent in everything that is not compatible with your physiology. Now, let's not say we're chasing shadows. If we can't find other obvious reasons for our sorry rates of chronic diseases, it would behoove us to seriously consider the dangers in our food and environment.

I have before me a formidably long list of familiar household chemicals designated by the U.S. Department of Agriculture as hazardous, but I'm not going to encumber you with them. We don't have to live scared. Just live smart.

There's just one more item I absolutely must discuss with you, because it is an area of much unwarranted complacency. That area is the pollution trapped inside your home. In trying to create the maximum in energy efficiency, the builder, with you in mind, has also created a near-impervious shell in which indoor pollution is trapped and poisons the inhabitants quietly and unnoticed but very effectively. Be informed that the effects of this pollution are not minor. They are subtle but can be deadly if not protected against. Millions are poisoned daily and nightly. The typical American home holds much higher concentrations of pollution than a smoggy city. Heating and cooking gas, kerosene appliances, fireplaces, air conditioning systems, aerosol sprays, insulating materials, tobacco smoke, and radiation are some of the sources of indoor pollution. You are strongly advised to see that the air in your home is exchanged periodically, even in cold weather. Try to develop a sense of the condition of the air in your home. Remember that the air is not going to jump up and ask to be changed. You're in charge.

Recently more experts are conscious of magnetic fields and their adverse effects on human beings. They seem to have concluded that all electrical equipment emits some harmful effects, even if only a little. Now, I'm not saying that you should give up your beloved microwave oven. Remember we both feel that life is to be enjoyed. However, we have given up our lovely electric blanket. But then, I'm a wet blanket.

We have spoken at length about how our bodies are polluted. Let us now discuss some methods by which we can purge pollution out of our bodies. There are numerous ramifications on this subject; so all cannot be covered in these few pages. I will discuss them briefly and refer you to the list of recommended reading in the Appendix.

Body trash is discharged through the bowels, urinary system, lungs, and skin.

Some 50 years ago Dr. Jacobus Rinse, a chemical engineer, had a heart attack. He refused to accept bypass surgery and instead experimented on his own to find a way he could remedy his condition. His efforts continued several years, during which time he had another heart attack. Characteristically he persevered and finally arrived at a formula of food supplements which he felt would clean out the calcified plaque in his coronary arteries. He took his formula for breakfast every morning and reportedly after six months was playing golf again without restrictions. He took up skiing at age 80. He helped many of his friends, and other people, to obtain similar results. Now the Rinse Formula is on the market and available in some health food stores. But should you care to make the concoction yourself, here is the formula. I suggest you make enough for a week or two and store it in the refrigerator.

The following amounts are for a week's supply and expressed in liquid measure (by volume).

3 ounces granulated lecithin
3 ounces raw wheat germ
3 ounces brewer's yeast, debittered preferred
10 ounces wheat bran
1 ounce bone meal
3 ounces raw sunflower seeds

Mix all ingredients.

Take two heaping table-spoonfuls of the mix for breakfast daily supplemented with:

1000 mg vitamin C
400 mg vitamin E
1 tbsp. good vegetable oil
2 garlic perles
2 or 3 kelp tablets
30 to 50 mg zinc
1 tablet potassium
1 tablet chromium
1 tablet multi-vitamin-mineral
1 cup milk (whole milk if you don't buy the cholesterol propaganda)

Dr. Rinse reportedly says he takes his "chicken feed" every morning and cares not what else he eats. I don't know whether he really said that, but you're smart enough to know we don't do things that way. You should observe all the rules of health to the best of your ability and patience. And that includes exercise. (Dr. Rinse strongly emphasizes exercise.) And that means getting your aerobics up for at least 20 minutes at least three times weekly. Well, you do want to clear up your arteries, don't you? We'll talk about exercise a bit later.

Then there's Robert Ford who says in his booklet "Fresh Food Versus Stale Food" that eating nothing but really fresh wholesome food and no junk at all will clear one's system of any arterial blockage. If conviction is any measure of the facts then Mr. ford is correct, because he appears extremely confident of his opinion. I am certain of one thing: His thoughts are absolutely in the right direction, but I don't really know how practically and effectively fresh food can do the job. And I also know that the effort can only benefit anyone conscientious enough to try it even if his arteries aren't completely cleared. Anyway, very few people, not even healthy ones, are free of crud. My conclusion: Do it. Success is a matter of degree.

Incidentally, here's an idea novel to most readers: I don't know how to appraise it but feel I should submit it to you as an interesting thought. You're on your own on this one. Mr. Ford advises against consumption of anything made of flour or meal of any kind. His reasoning is that the fineness of the particles allows them to penetrate the intestinal walls and bypass the filtering process. You may have heard of the DEAMOF (Don't eat anything made of flour.) diet I read about some 40 years ago.

No treatise on internal cleanliness can be complete without a discussion of fasting. The merits of fasting must be recognized when one notes that the practice is recorded throughout the pages of history and in all areas of the world. Fasting is resting the digestive functions, but that is not the whole story. When your body is relieved of the responsibility of digesting and assimilating food, it is free to do what it always wants to do: clean house. When a conscientious homemaker gets a vacation or a weekend away from her outside job, she tends to want to clean house. Your body does the same. If you keep feeding your face and stomach without a let-up, your body may never get a chance to get its house clean and the trash keeps building up and gives rise to free radicals, and you know that excessive free radicals are gremlins we can do without. The result is of course a sick body.

Not only does your body try to clean out the garbage left over from last night's dinner; given the chance it also digs out and purges old sludge deposited and stored from times past. On long serious fasts, years-old crud is sometimes pulled out. At the end of such fasts, the body, while usually much underweight, is for the most part clean and free of any chronic disease. It is well known that prisoners of war who have been starved skinny come home with clean arteries.

If you are conscientious enough to want to fast, numerous good books on the subject are available. There are an endless number of ways to fast, some of which are very easy and conservative, like a one-day fruit- or vegetable-juice fast, for example.

I feel that almost everybody can benefit from fasting, even those who feel they are clean. Probably everybody has some blockage of the coronary arteries. Symptoms of arteriosclerosis don't occur until the arteries are about 75 percent blocked, or even more. Your body is very forgiving — up to a point. When it can tolerate no more of your transgressions, down you go.

If you're looking for a controversy you're in the right place. But the controversy is not warranted and not a true one. It is powered by the love of that green stuff. Tired of that explanation? I am too. Sorry, but that is par for the course. Let's just say that the controversy is a synthetic one, not unlike the rest of their drugs. Big Med says that chelation is still experimental and therefore does not recognize it as a legitimate treatment. Very few insurance companies will pay for chelation services, and I don't have to tell you about the interlocking relationships between these two industries.

Chelation is pronounced kee-lay-shun and is derived from the Greek "khele," which means claw, because the chelating agent claws at the calcified plaque and pulls it out of the arteries, passing it out of the body mostly through the kidneys and bladder. It is administered intravenously, the patient typically sitting in an easy chair and receiving about a pint of an amino acid dripped into his veins over about three-and-a-half hours. The entire treatment is time-consuming and typically comprises 30 to 40 sessions, at the rate of two or three per week, the number required depending on the severity of the patient's condition. It is comparatively very safe and allows the patient to simultaneously converse, read, or watch television. After-treatment activities are free of restrictions.

What about costs? Treatments are typically $75 to $100 per session and so a series of 30 sessions would cost $3000 to $4000, not quite as much as the $40,000-or-so setback for a coronary bypass, and there's the big reason why chelation is still "experimental" and "controversial."

This "experiment" and "controversy" have been going on for well over 50 years, and some doctors have made their observations and drawn their conclusions long ago, and have helped thousands of patients regain their health with clean blood vessels throughout their entire bodies, relieving not only blocked arteries but also a myriad of other miseries, arthritis very much included. I have seen the dramatic results for myself — all of this while avoiding the risk of the scalpel, which addresses only the coronary arteries, and the accompanying drugs that are so detrimental to health, not to mention the financial cost. But not to fret. The laws of balance are still at work, and what cost the patient and all the insurance policyholders suffer accrues to and is enjoyed by Big Medi$in. So all is not lost.

While chelation treatment for atherosclerosis is still "experimental" and "controversial," it has been since as far back as 1942 the standard protocol for the treatment of lead and mercury poisonings and poisonings of other metals. And, lo and behold, insurance pays for it. Why the inconsistency? Is there some difference somewhere between the harmful effects of lead and calcium? Of course there's a difference, but the difference you're probably thinking about is not the reason for the difference in the insurance treatment, and why chelation of calcium, also a metal, is still "experimental" and "controversial." Chelation of lead and mercury from the body does not rob the surgeon of his "livelihood." Big Medi$in cannot justify their high-handedness, but with their formidable financial and political clout they can just stand there bold-faced and hold their ground. After all, this is the U.S. of A., and we cannot legislate morality, let alone successfully combat illegal acts of injustice.

There can be no doubt of the effectiveness of chelation. It's scientifically sound. It has achieved spectacular success. How can anyone, aside from reasons of finance, prefer to have only his coronary arteries reamed out when he can have the same cleaning benefits for the arteries to his legs, arms, internal organs, brain, and skeletal joints? If a patient is senile because of an insufficiency of blood to his brain before his bypass operation, he will still be senile after the bypass. Too, the benefits of the bypass are notoriously short-lived. My friend has had two bypass operations, the first one a triple and the second a quintuple.

Ted Rosema, M.D., of Raleigh, N.C., says of chelation: "I do this and take the flak I get for doing it for only one reason, and that is the benefit I see for my patients. It's the first time in my 25 years of medical practice that I've actually seen patients get better rather than go downhill." Does this also say quite a lot about all the other aspects of conventional medicine?

If you would like more information on chelation, including names of chelation practitioners near you, write:

The American Academy of Medical Preventics
8383 Wilshire Blvd., Suite 922
Beverly Hills, CA 90211
Telephone (213) 878-1234

An enlightening book on the subject: "The Chelation Way," by Dr. Morton Walker.

The purpose of chelation is to clean out the arteries, but clean arteries aren't the only requisite for internal cleanliness. The eliminative system, in plain words the guts, needs to be allowed to fulfill its important function without the interference of crud. But unfortunately in our society the overwhelming majority of us are walking cesspools. Is it any wonder that colorectal cancer is on the increase? The well-known Dr. Harvey W. Kellog said, "Of the 22,000 operations I have personally performed, I have never seen a single normal colon."

We must remember to consider the age-old advice to drink plenty of good, clean water. It is excellent advice. Dehydration is one of our serious "diseases" and gives rise to many further ills. You would do well to drink six to eight glasses of good water daily.

When you sport a clean pretty pink tongue, when you have two (yes, two) easy, productive, comparatively odor-free bowel movements daily, when your urine is almost colorless, when you get up in the morning with a clean-tasting mouth, you'll know you're well on your way to good health. But of course how well you progress along that path will depend a lot on how well you fulfill the other requisites for health.

Near the beginning of this chapter on health, we discussed intestinal flora, dental fillings, and dental root canals. These three subjects were placed there to attract your especial attention, not only because they concern a goodly portion of our population but also because they have not received their deserved share of attention from health advisors. They are a very important part of the discussion at hand, and so I strongly suggest that you go back and be sure to give due consideration to the thoughts presented. Whether or not you buy the rationales, they will at least provide useful exercise for your mind.

NUTRITION

Because of the large areas of overlap between internal cleanliness and nutrition, some repetition will be inevitable. But this is okay, because I cannot assume any order in which you will read this book, or even that you will read all of it.

Should you read this section before or without reading the preceding one, I would not want you to be in want of relevant information.

A former Regional Superintendent of Inspection Services, Food and Drug Division, Department of Health and Welfare, Vancouver, British Columbia, wrote and published a booklet entitled "Stop Killing Yourself and Begin to Live." This in part is what he said:

"There is a crying need for that manner of education that teaches the average man and woman how to be well, strong and full of energy and endurance, and how to preserve their health through living on a non-disease-producing diet. By teaching them that the cause of practically all disease is a poisoned blood stream resulting from the popular diet of unnatural devitalized food. (Sic)

"There is, perhaps, no field of education more sorely neglected than that of human nutrition. People are dying, literally, by the millions because of the great lack of information relative to the food they consume..."

Notice again, above, the position formerly held by the author of those words. Few people are better qualified to speak on this subject. I had better take back those words, because actually many people are so qualified. But for some reason they cannot or will not say what they know. This country is just too darned loaded with political deterrents to freedom of speech. Legally we have our First Amendment, but it's no panacea; we still cannot freely speak our minds. Can you imagine hearing an American cabinet member say something similar to what that Canadian official said? Hah!

Recognizing the gravity of the dangers we now face so complacently, I would be remiss, indeed guilty, if I neglected to write this letter to you.

Behold the contrast. In America the Beautiful many of the people who know better say that diet is not important, and those who don't speak those stupid words and are in position to take the bull by the horns turn the other way and neglect to try to improve our sorry lot. Lord, forgive them, even though they do know what evil they do and neglect to do what they ought.

So much for neglect, disloyalty, infidelity, treachery, greed, selfishness, self-service, insincerity, dishonesty, and just plain old evil.

A question often asked is, "What should one eat to be healthy?" To that I respond that it is more practical to first discuss what we should not eat, because those foods are easier to categorize and omission of them from our diets will automatically restrict us to good food.

For the sake of simplicity let us use the term "junk food" or "junk" to identify what we should not eat. Not all food is black or white. Much of it is gray in varying shades. On the premise that too stringent an attitude toward food would tend to discourage the aspirant, and therefore conversely that some compromise would tend to enhance the probability of success by making the goals more attainable, you should decide how demanding you should be on yourself in your pursuit of health. And that brings us to the question, "What is junk food?" Let us generalize and then allow you to decide to what degree you should adhere to our definitions.

Junk food is that which is no longer in a natural state, the state that existed shortly after that food was presented to us by Mother. I say "shortly after" because stale food, even though not corrupted by man, has been modified by time and is no longer in its natural state. The merits of the natural state were discussed in the last section.

277

In the interest of perspective, in an attempt at completeness, and at the expense of being very verbose, I will rattle off a whole string of adjectives to describe junk food: processed, denatured, refined, overcooked, devitalized, foodless, adulterated, fragmented, overripe, fractionalized, manufactured, synthetic, stale, rancid, dead, rotten, unnatural, altered, modified, embellished, improved, enriched, molded, smoked, perverted, converted, irradiated, preserved, salted, seasoned, charred, pickled, frozen, cured, corned, blackened, fried, sugared, artificially flavored, artificially colored, chemically fertilized, reconstituted, concentrated, chemically sprayed, canned, sweetened, homogenized, hydrogenated, stabilized, emulsified. Mercy! But notice that I spared you your cherished barbecue. I'll leave that one up to you as with the other bad words above. In short, any food characterized by any of those adjectives should have no place in your body. But you notice that I have my tongue in my cheek. And I use that word "should" loosely, as, again, you know how you want to run your program.

Though the deleterious effects of junk food were discussed at length in the last section, let's briefly summarize them here. When food loses its natural, or complete, state, it loses some of its nutritive value. But that's not so bad. What's worse is that the factors in the food that have lost their usefulness and therefore cannot be converted to blood and tissue are now excess baggage, trash, garbage. Still that doesn't sound so bad. "The body is designed to dispose of that stuff, isn't it? So what's the big deal? Everybody eats junk all day long, every day, and they're getting along. In fact most people look pretty good." Hold it. You're speaking on an erroneous assumption. People may look okay to you but they're not always so. The great Life Force is so faithful, gracious, and forgiving that it holds us up to the best of its ability until our reserve is exhausted. And then you know what happens. Look at our young people and their junk. Look at the growing cancer and suicide rates among them. They will be sicker than our generation. Will it be in spite of Big Medi$in or because of Big Medi$in?

The Life Force tries its best to purge the garbage, also known as toxemia, or poison. So far, so good. But here comes the difficulty. Our modern diet is so full of junk that our bodies are hard-put to get rid of it. Even a century-and-a-half has not been nearly enough time to build up the additional ability required to purge the huge amount of junk we have added to our diets only recently. "Sure, people get sick. That's only natural. But they get well again and still live 70 or 80 years." Yes, but do you notice how feeble and decrepit some of them get before they finally run out of gas? To many of them "life is just not worth living anymore." They're stuck in a chair in a corner and nobody talks to them. Who wants to talk with them when they're so out-of-it? Hey, don't you scoff at those old folks. If you don't take charge of yourself now you could some day be one of them. If you're satisfied with dying prematurely at 80 after a lingering incapacitating illness, I guess it's your right. But don't wait too long to change your mind.

The backlog of junk produces free radicals which attack our cells and make us old and dead before our time. I said "us" just to be polite. I don't intend to be old before my time. After all, I've got 30 or 40 years to go yet. With proper care man should be able to live past the century mark in good health. This is not mere conjecture. In some remote areas of the world, notably the Himalayan country of Hunza, such a healthy condition exists. The men there play polo into their nineties and also father babies at that age. They reportedly have no police force, nor do they need any. As to be expected, the Hunzakuts live with nature and try their best to avoid the influences of the "advanced" nations. Smart people. Healthy people. No police.

The Hunzakuts are not the only such people. Similar populations have been found in all parts of the world. Though widely separated geographically, they all share the same lifestyle: They live close to nature and have not been cursed with the blessings of "civilization."

In 1979 I visited the little island republic of Nauru, situated in the vast Pacific Ocean. I walked around that island in about 30 minutes. How is it that such a little island is a republic? Because its inhabitants are rich and dependent on no one. Many, many years ago, before man lived there, Nauru was home to a huge population of sea birds. Over the years, their droppings, known in agriculture as guano, accumulated and eventually amounted to huge volumes. A by-product of fish-eating birds, it was extremely rich, especially in phosphorus. It was only a matter of time when some enterprising entity discovered the rich bounty and decided to mine what is now known as phosphate. One might well call it phosphate ore, as owing to the many years of existence it no longer resembles bird droppings.

One result of the commercialization of Nauru's phosphate is that, I have read, the per capita income of its inhabitants is greater than that of the United States. These people who only a few years ago were typical island natives living off the land and sea, were now affluent and to a great extent living in the ways of the "advanced" nations. I could not help being impressed by the universal presence of soft-drink cans and candy wrappers, both on the ground and in the shops. When I mentioned this piteous condition to a middle-aged gentleman who looked to be a tourist, he told me apparently on good authority that about 35 percent of the local population were diabetic. How tragic, I thought, and wondered whether the remainder of them were hypoglycemic. Perhaps it is too optimistic to hope the trend has been reversed. Haunted by such a sorrowful statistic, I wrote to Nauru, specifically the Director of Health Services, and asked for further statistics on the health situation there. Unfortunately I received no reply. All I can do is hope, without much hope, that my self-appointed statistician was not correct in his report to me, and that the Director of Health Services was not himself diabetic and in too poor a condition to dig up the statistics if he had kept any at all.

I lived and worked as a civil servant for the U.S. Navy on Guam for fourteen years, from 1966 to 1980. Being health-oriented, I noticed the dietary behavior of the Guamanians, known ethnically as Chamorros. They had become thoroughly Americanized, having begun their transition after World War II, when they became officially the U.S. Territory of Guam. They often proudly referred to themselves as Guam, U.S.A. The population comprised, when I lived there, about one-half Chamorros and Filipinos and one-half "Statesiders," which included civilians and military service personnel. As life there was influenced almost completely by military and commercial activity, the local population was well integrated into the American way of life. And of course you know what I'm about to say; that they consumed their share, and considerably more, of soft drinks, doughnuts and other sweet pastries, hamburgers and fries. It was an accepted practice among some locals to feed their babies cola drinks in a nippled milk bottle. In the early seventies McDonald's built the chain's largest store worldwide on Guam. Their reception surpassed

281

expectations. And of course you already know what happened to the physical health of the people of Guam.

In 1992, I wrote to Dr. Robert E. Haddock, Territorial Epidemiologist on Guam, and asked for statistics on the history of health among the Chamorro population on Guam. Below are the data Dr. Haddock sent me:

	1947	1988	Increase
Chamorro population of Guam	48,336	129,306	168%
# of deaths due to diabetes	1	26	2500%
# of deaths due to cancer	6	91	1417%
# of deaths due to heart disease	8	128	1500%

So it's Nauru all over again. Cumulatively deaths due to these three degenerative diseases (symptoms) increased 16 times faster than the increase in population between 1947 and 1988, the period of adjustment to the American way. Of course the change in diet is not the whole story. Largely the local people work in government and business offices and have forgotten how to fish and farm.

The notion of diet's being a major cause of adverse conditions of the body or a help in remedying adverse conditions is generally scoffed at, in varying degrees, not only by Big Medi$in but also by many people at large. We know that the medical gods wield heavy influence on society's attitudes, but could it also be that we hold food sacrosanct and refuse to attribute any adverse results to diet because undisciplined eating is one of life's greatest pleasures?

Are the farmers, grocers, and doctors the villains and we the victims? That's not half true. We are the true villains who victimize ourselves. We have control over what we buy and eat and therefore what the business people produce and provide for us. We also have control over what services we seek from our doctors and therefore what services our doctors render us. A man with a warehouseful of profitable drugs isn't going to turn away customers who come to his door. By Ned, if you don't want the man to drug you, stay out of his office. If you don't want to be jabbed with a needle and pumped full of chemicals keep your sleeves down and your pants up. Ultimately you are responsible for what these people do to you. Exercise your options and responsibilities.

"Society is so horrible now. Crime is rampant and out of control. I wonder why." A healthy mind does not produce crime. Hardened criminals have been reformed with experimental diets. Mental health and physical health are inextricably mutually integrated.

Have we been eminently successful in maintaining a healthy and happy society? Would it be absolutely absurd to suggest that perhaps health would help? But we cannot depend on government to determine what we stuff our faces with. We must do that for ourselves. If we would have a better world to live in, we as a society must venture beyond what comes naturally and be governed more by, and with, our God-given brains than by our creature pleasures. We would then be exchanging a few minutes of superficial pleasure for a lifetime of physical and spiritual health.

Let us return now to the original question, "What should one eat to be healthy?" A simple but accurate answer would be, "Just the converse of the foods described above as being inferior by virtue of being in an unnatural state." But that's

283

a bit flippant. So let's expand on the subject. First we will do for the superior foods what we did for the inferior. So here are a few adjectives used to describe the foods favorable to our health: natural, whole, complete, fresh, living, wholesome, vibrant, unprocessed, unrefined, undefiled, pure, live, organically grown.

There is no shortage of literature to tell you which of the good foods are better for you. Rather than do this and nettle your mind with specifics, I prefer to say this: All foods in their natural state and established as being edible are good foods and should be duly appreciated. Read an article on potatoes and you'll discover what a great food they are. Ditto for cabbage, rutabaga, radishes, apples. Each food has its own unique merits. We need not find out which is better. Rather we should strive to be sure we get a good variety of foods in our diet. We avail ourselves of this variety by enlisting the help of our five senses. If you have a sixth one, like intuition, use it too. Try to eat as many colors as you can. Make rainbow salads. Enjoy a wide range of flavors. Even bitter vegetables tell us they're full of valuable minerals, not only the ones dietitians tell us about but perhaps also some we have never consciously discovered. Go for contrasting fragrances and aromas too. Ah, garlic! The onion and the rose smell different because they're storehouses of different nutrients. The fruit of the rose is the second richest known natural source of vitamin C. Do you like the audible crack of the first bite into a fresh healthy red apple? But isn't it also comforting to feel the gentle pear squishing in your mouth? How about some nice golden squash? The mealiness of a good baked potato is made more enjoyable by the contrast of a young red beet. Crunchiness in fruits and vegetables tells us that we're eating fresh foods.

Of course you know I'm not referring to the crispness of fried or burnt foods.

Let's get a bit more specific and discuss the parts of foods. What a waste to discard the core of a head of cabbage, an apple or a pear, the root of celery, the outer green leaves of leafy vegetables (if they haven't been sprayed with commercial chemicals), the tops and skins of many fruits and vegetables. These parts all offer variety in nutrients. Only the threat of toxic chemical treatments discourages us from using them. But this threat should not instill in us an irrational fear. The converse of smelling the roses of life is to not unduly fear every little threat. If you make an overall effort to keep your system clean and thus your immune system durable, you should be better able to tolerate the hazards of a few toxic sprays, an occasional cup of coffee, an after-dinner mint chocolate.

Inhabitants of the less affluent countries make considerable use of parts of plants we routinely discard, notably blossoms and seeds of the squash family and the young leaves of vines. The buds of the day lily are a major and relished food item.

As a rule, the seeds of food plants are bursting with rich nutrients. After all, a seed is an agent of reproduction and stores the nutrients required for the new life to follow. Incidentally some health advisors are not in favor of eating seedless varieties of fruits, the reason given being that they are deficient in manganese, a valuable trace element. Too, they have no seeds to eat and therefore are further short of goodies.

Variety is to be sought not only within categories of foods but also between, or among, the categories. We should try to strike a balance by eating fruits, vegetables (including sprouts), whole-grain cereals, seeds, nuts, and (Oh-oh) animal products. I'm slightly ambivalent about animal products but on balance in favor of them. They will be discussed soon.

The benefits offered by the different categories of foods differ considerably and are substantial in every one of them. Volumes have been written on this subject and so I will not try to re-invent the health book. I'll only say that you should remember to adequately include all the categories of foods in your diet, because differences in nutrients are greater between categories than within the individual categories.

If you consume a wide variety of natural foods and shun the junk, your efforts at health will be considerably simplified in that you will not have to excessively worry about free radicals and antioxidants. Our lives have already been rendered too complex and demanding. Let's not make health a chore.

We have discussed free radicals and antioxidants in the previous pages but I must direct your attention to them again. I highly recommend that you go back to the section just before this one, the one on internal cleanliness, and contemplate especially pycnogenol and kombucha.

Here's a little food for creative thought, an exercise in questioning conventional wisdom and in thinking for yourself: I don't think roasted peanuts deserve as much respect as they are honored with. "Roasted" peanuts are fried peanuts. Some labels are even honest enough to tell you that (Read labels!). Even "dry-roasted" peanuts and those roasted in the shell are fried. The flesh of raw peanuts are white and soft. After roasting they are brown and crunchy. What made them brown and crunchy? Being rich in oil, they have been internally fried in their own oil. I'm not saying roasted peanuts are bad, but we should recognize that they are fried.

Now, what about animal products? I don't think there's a pat answer here. I am aware that many vegetarians and meat eaters are well convinced of their opinions, but let me explain. Idealistically speaking, meaning that if we all were in superb physical condition, we would all react to foods exactly alike. Nobody would have allergies or individual idiosyncrasies. Unfortunately, most of us fall short of physical perfection and so differ from one another in an infinite number of ways. As is often said, one man's meat is another's poison.

Having contemplated this age-old controversy, I must admit that the vegetarians seem to have a slight edge on theory. I have even tried to be one of them but it just wouldn't work for me. I would down a huge salad and a big platter of potatoes, beans, and broccoli and still be hungry. My stomach would feel full to its limit but my body would be crying for energy. I tried several times over the years to subsist on vegetarian meals but just couldn't do it. Perhaps being a hypoglycemic has something to do with the difference between the vegetarians and me. Being hungry after a big meal wasn't merely being hungry; it was downright traumatic. I was nervous and shaky. Having given the effort a sincere go, I have decided to quit worrying about it and enjoy my medium-rare porterhouse steaks, prime rib, barbecued ribs, lobster, shrimp, oysters, clams, crabs, sashimi, swimming fish, opihi, wana, haukiuki, poki, kalua pig, caviar, squab, pheasant, turkey, Peking duck, eggs, Limburger cheese, bleu cheese, Monterey jack, and whatever other good stuff lands on my platter. No, I don't trim off all the visible fat and I don't skin my chicken. You too some day will find out the fallacy of the Great Cholesterol Scare.

287

Soviet Georgia probably has a new name now, but anyway, it reportedly has more centenarians among its people than any other area in the world. Sorry, but the people there eat large amounts of fatty meats and whole milk products. Apparently sugar and white flour are still the champion troublemakers.

On balance I feel the vegetarians are on the right track — but only for themselves. If you can subsist on veggies, and want to do so, go to it. But be sure to do it right. Without meats you will be depriving your body of some very essential building materials. Too many vegetarians look like vegetarians. Learn from the experts, the ones whose success is evidenced by good health. The result will be cleaner inners and much less garbage for your physiology to worry with.

"The Milk of Human Kindness Is Not Pasteurized." That is the title of a book by William Campbell Douglass, M.D. As an MD who has not allowed himself to be fettered by the Establishment, Dr. Douglass warrants the respect not only of health-minded people but also of all who take human values seriously. (His book is listed in the Appendix.) He says so much so well that I feel a bit foolish discussing his subject. But on the premise that you may not read this book, let's have a brief discussion of milk here.

It has often been said that cow's milk is for baby cows or baby bulls and not fit for human consumption. How valid that statement is, is another heavy controversy. But let's not try to resolve it, as it would be a moot effort, anyway. People love milk and we cannot begin to stop the flow of the millions of gallons all over this big country. So the most sensible thing to do is to present a few salient facts as I know them. This discussion also may be moot, as, given the political aspects of milk, there may not be very much you can do with the information given below. But let's offer you the information anyway, for whatever value it may hold for you.

Goat's milk is far superior to cow's milk in probably all aspects. It's much more nourishing. It's naturally homogenized. It's much less allergenic and causes much less mucus. But if you don't have a goat or live near a goat farm, the health food store is probably your only source but it probably will be pasteurized and devoid of some of its original nutrients. More people worldwide drink goat's milk than cow's. The Myenburg Goat Milk Company of Santa Barbara, CA, distributes powdered goat's milk nationally.

Certified raw cow's milk, or other clean raw milk, is far superior by any practical measure to pasteurized and homogenized. Pasteurization kills the all-important enzymes and some vitamins and renders the product less digestible and assimilable. The milk is now incomplete food and adds more free radicals to the system.

The following information has been voiced by several health researchers and I consider it the most important datum I'm offering here on milk: Homogenization of milk is a major cause of heart disease. The reduced size of the fat globules, they say, allows them to penetrate the intestinal walls, enter the bloodstream undigested, and contribute to atherosclerosis. Given the almost-universal respect accorded that enjoyable white stuff, I can easily imagine that you will have to take the above information with several large grains of salt. I don't blame you, but at least I have told you.

I find it pretty difficult to bad-mouth milk, because I enjoy it immensely myself. Homogenization makes it taste so rich, and milk more than any other food seems to deliver the energy to my body immediately after being swallowed. Oh, the frustrations of life!

But you don't have to capitulate to the health nuts. If you love milk as I do, you may want to share my philosophy: I say to myself, "You take pretty good care of yourself. Your immune system is top-notch. You minimize the free radicals in your body. So what the heck! Be kind to yourself and enjoy some milk now and then." But don't think you can rationalize like this any time your fancy strikes you if you indulge in too many other vices. You have to qualify.

This is for Californians only: If you share my sentiments on milk and would like to give your children certified raw milk, here is some information for you: The Alta-Dena Certified Dairy distributes high-quality certified raw milk in California only. But they distribute nationwide other products made from certified raw milk. Their telephone number is (800) 535-1369.

More controversy, anyone? The next hot subject is eggs. The odds are that to you it's a hands-down, cut-and-dried case. Egg yolks contain cholesterol and therefore are bad for you. Well, maybe yes and maybe no. You've heard the negative side of the story maybe 200 times, in the form of direct statements, innuendoes, or allusions. So let's look at the other side. There's no doubt that egg yolks contain a lot of cholesterol, but one analyst says that yolks also have abundant lecithin, eight times the amount required to metabolize the cholesterol contained.

I have seen a two-in-one graph showing the decline in the consumption of eggs in recent years and the increase in heart attacks. The two lines form an "X." If eggs cause atherosclerosis, why does the rate of heart attacks keep rising while the consumption of eggs keeps declining? One must wonder.

Have you heard or read of the 88-year-old man who at the time of the report had eaten between 20 and 30 eggs every day for the last 15 years and had a serum cholesterol reading varying between 150 and 200 mg/dl? I read of him in two respectable articles and heard it on TV.

Dr. H.W. Holdenby gave some of his patients five eggs per day for a period of time with no change in their average cholesterol readings.

A hundred men were each fed 18 eggs per week for six months and their serum cholesterol readings were lower at the end of the experiment than at the start.

Having learned something about the causal relationship between dietary fat and serum cholesterol and having seen so many "conventional wisdoms" flushed down the tube, I never did buy the current one about fat and eggs, 260 million Americans notwithstanding. Anyway, I never did deprive myself of any morsel of fat I took a fancy to. And I consume roughly a dozen eggs per week. But how are my coronary arteries? The Mayo Clinic told me a couple years ago that they were in good shape. And just this morning as I write this, my doctor looked at the laboratory report of my tests and exclaimed, "I wish everybody had your kind of circulation. I mean everybody, young and old."

Now, I'm not telling you that fat is good for you. I'm saying that I enjoy smelling the roses and also the crispy fat right out of the oven. But I indulge in these little vices because I have taken measures to fortify myself against an occasional misdemeanor.

By the way, if you eat eggs and are fortunate enough to have a choice, try to find "country eggs," or real eggs, meaning those which are laid by happy hens who are serviced by a rooster and who scratch around in the dirt and eat real food from Mother Earth. Analysis has shown a considerable difference between them and the manufactured ones.

Moreover, what other wholesome protein and fat can you buy for 60 cents a pound, or even a dollar a pound?

Even assuming that dietary fat does increase serum cholesterol, which I doubt, its effect is next to nothing when compared to that of sugar and white flour products. I keep wondering why our establishment of health do-gooders harp so much on the supposed evil of fat and say next to nothing about the real culprits. Sugar and flour produce much more serum cholesterol than does a little fat, not to say anything about the tons of free radicals, the ultimate destroyers of health.

A few additional comments on nutrition:

Nutrition isn't only the selection of good foods. It's also the avoidance of junk foods, the maintenance of internal cleanliness.

Perishable foods are far superior to preserved foods. They are perishable because their nutrient quality attracts microbial life. Preserved foods are resistant to decay because they contain elements inimical to life. Germs can't thrive on them and neither can you; neither should you try to. Select fresh perishable foods and consume them before our little friends get to them.

"If you have a balanced diet you don't need food supplements. Supplements are just the bait used by the quacks to separate you from your money." How many times have you heard that one? And you know who's drumming that same old song. Sadly, many people will say, after reading that advice, "The doctor says we don't need supplements. He says they're a big rip-off." The doctors' big word here is "if." But the fact is, it's well nigh impossible to sustain a balanced diet in today's world. But "if" you did have a balanced diet, should you take food supplements? Well, let's see. Does your balanced diet consist of mostly natural food and very few junk foods? Do you have a good mental attitude with a minimum of emotional stresses? Do you exercise enough to keep your physiology durable and well toned? Do you get enough rest? Is your environment comparatively free of industrialized air? Is your drinking water pure, free of chlorine and fluorides? Is your home pollution-free? Do you avoid hair sprays, other high-tech cosmetics, and volatile liquids? Yes? Then perhaps you don't need food supplements. Or, if you couldn't care less whether you're healthy or sick, perhaps you don't need supplements.

"It's so unnatural to take things to supplement one's diet. If Nature intended for us to have supplements she would have grown some for us." You're right. And she does grow a lot of it for us, and gave us brains to enable us to use her gifts intelligently to counteract our unnatural culture. Intelligently studied and used, supplements can be an exceedingly gratifying blessing, a positive measure without side effects, which is more than can be said of drugs. They are not simply vitamins and minerals anymore, but a very bona fide health science. The guesswork has been all but eliminated. Most of the supplements are simply natural foods known to be rich in certain beneficial factors and concentrated into convenient tablets or capsules. The dehydration required for successful packaging and marketing concentrates the foods and renders them more effective in their functions. Natural food supplements restore and maintain homeostasis as they nourish the body. Do we need food supplements? Especially with the recent advances made in natural nutrition I'd say they are a great blessing and enhance the quality of life. If you've been taking supplements but don't notice the benefits, it could be because (1) you're eating junk food to nullify the benefits of your supplements, (2) you're not taking the right supplements, or (3) your body hasn't "caught up" yet, meaning your supplements are still working on your deficits, and when they get you up to par you should feel the benefits. Your faith and patience will reward you.

While a balanced diet of wholesome food is a major concern, many of the supplemental health products on the market offer special benefits to enhance health. If you are not familiar with them their sheer number and variety could be daunting and cause you to ignore them altogether. I've been there too but now, after years of study and experience, feel I know pretty well what's what. By and large, the natural products most widely promoted by the reputable health food purveyors are valid and beneficial. This dependability is enhanced by the considerable competition among the many quality suppliers today.

I will list and describe below a few food supplements which have proven themselves with their performance and their popularity:

Ginkgo biloba: Extracted from the leaves of a tree which is said to be the oldest living tree species, a survivor from before the ice age. It is extremely popular in Europe, where more that 20 million people reportedly take it. The Chinese have used it for centuries to preserve youth and vitality. It cleans out blood vessels, especially those leading to the brain, thus forestalling or preventing senility.

Saw palmetto: Promotes health of men's and women's reproductive systems. Reportedly effective in treating prostatitis.

Shark cartilage: A comparatively recent discovery showing impressive promise in the treatment of cancer.

Notwithstanding my usual disdain for specific cures, test results are convincing.

Spirulina and Chlorella: Algae products rich in several nutrients, especially protein and chlorophyll, a great natural antioxidant. These two great products are cultivated mostly in the Far East.

Garlic and onions: Known as the king and queen of vegetables. Rich in nutrients and antioxidants. Garlic, especially, is widely hailed as an antibiotic. (As I have indicated, I'm not wild about antibiotics.)

L-carnitine: Strengthens heart action.

Coenzyme Q10, also known as CQ10: An antioxidant enzyme produced by the body but not in sufficient supplies to nullify the effects of the artificially abundant quantities of free radicals produced in today's culture. It is a popular item in the health foods market. A popular claim made for CQ10 is that in severe periodontal problems where the only remedy seems to be wholesale extraction of teeth, CQ10 can save the day — and the teeth. It is said that 30 mg of the enzyme per day for three weeks are on record as having saved one patient's teeth.

Pycnogenol: A very important supplement that I suggest you take very seriously. There's no doubt about its unusual value in human health, but rather than haranguing you with a lengthy repetition, I suggest you review it in the last section, "Inner Cleanliness."

Kombucha, or Mushroom tea: What I've just said about pycnogenol applies with equal force to kombucha.

Bee pollen and Royal jelly: Two super foods extremely rich in a wide variety of nutrients. You can buy these with confidence.

Ginseng: A mysterious but effective supplement that has gained rapidly increasing recognition and popularity in recent years. The reason for its effectiveness thus far seems to be a riddle even to health researchers, but apparently nobody can naysay it.

DHEA: The initials of a substance with a long jawbreaker of a name which few people, except the specialists, know and which thus is not a convenient name to use. The initials serve the purpose of identification very well. DHEA is heralded by some as one of the very most important health discoveries of our time. It is referred to as the "mother of enzymes," meaning it enhances the action of other enzymes. Keep your eyes and ears open and try to learn more about it.

Colloidal silver: Another supplement excitedly heralded for its effectiveness in promoting health. Primarily it is an antibiotic and has done wonders for many people. But as you probably know by now, antibiotics don't excite me much except in a negative way. They're sometimes good for the individual in the short run, but society doesn't benefit in the long run by the use of antibiotics by anybody.

While we're looking at examples of food supplements, let's look at examples of good foods and bad foods:

Some of the Best Foods	Some of the Worse Foods
Fruits, melons	White or brown sugar
Leafy greens	White flour
Root vegetables	Sweet pastries
Legumes	Cakes, pies
Garlic	Candies
Onions	Commercial ice cream
Sprouts	Cola drinks
Parsley	Soda pop
Squashes	Coffee

Herb teas	Chocolate
Avocado	French fries
Whole grains	Lard, bacon, ham,
Brown rice	and other cured meats
Wheat germ	Potato chips,
Wheat bran	other salted snacks
Nuts, seeds	Sausage
Yogurt	Soup mixes, prepared
Buttermilk	Oleomargarine, other
Brewer's yeast	hydrogenated fats
Eggs ("country")	Pickles
Fish, fowl	Alcoholic drinks
Meats (moderate amounts)	Preserved foods
	Synthetic foods

As a rule, beverages should not be taken shortly before, during, or shortly after meals. Taken shortly before or after, they dilute the digestive juices of the stomach and thus hinder digestion. Taken during meals, they tend to wash the food down and deprive it of saliva and its digestive enzymes, not to mention inadequacy of chewing. If you feel the need for more liquid, try salads as a replacement.

If discipline in eating and drinking poses a problem for you, the following strategy might help you:

If you want to sprinkle more salt on your dinner but feel you shouldn't, tough it out without yielding until the last couple of bites. Then sprinkle a little salt and enjoy the end of your meal. The aftertaste will remain for a while and the deprivation will be easier on you. The modicum of self respect you gain will be an added dividend.

If you must drink ice tea, try using a smaller glass, drink it plain until the last gulp or two, then add a teaspoon or less of sugar. He who laughs last laughs best. Of course, if you can do without the tea or sugar, so much the better. Self respect tastes better than sugar any time. I guess.

The same strategy can be used in an infinite number of similar situations.

I will tell you about a good mental game you may want to adopt for yourself. At home in our freezer door we keep a five-ounce drinking glass full of ice cubes. Whenever we get a Coke attack we can't handle, we fill that little glass full of the Real Thing. We drink about two ounces of the bad stuff but get the satisfaction of downing five full ounces. We keep telling ourselves that, anyway.

MIND and SPIRIT

In this section we will discuss not only the interrelation between physical and mental health, but also mental health for its own sake, for mental health is health too.

Were I to designate one aspect of spirit to be the greatest asset to a health program, it would be gratitude for our wondrous bodies and minds. If you have studied to any extent the workings of nature, not only man's but of all life, you understand what I'm trying to express. Recognizing the abundant beauty and profound blessings of our world I often notice myself to be in wordless prayer to our loving Creator. Healthful living is for me a spiritual activity. Appreciation and respect for my body and mind help me to maintain the tender loving care I give them, and this of course enhances my health.

Here's how gratitude can be a great blessing to you: Be consciously grateful for all the workings of your body and mind, even your symptoms, your pains, colds, nausea, fever, mucus, swollen lymph nodes. Be fascinated by your body's responses to whatever ails you. Don't bemoan your symptoms, for they are a part of healing. Marvel at their workings. Watch and enjoy the regeneration of tissue. Cut your mind and spirit in on the healing project. The insight you gain will make you a better steward of your body and mind.

"Do you not know that your body is a temple of the Holy Spirit within you, which you have from God? You are not your own; you were bought with a price. So glorify God in your body." "Whether you eat or drink or whatever you do, do all to the glory of God."

— 1 Cor. 6:19-20; 10:31

In all that you contemplate and do, invite your spirit team to participate, for they are your source of wisdom.

Another extremely valuable asset in a health program is interpersonal compatibility, especially in a marriage or other serious partnership. It can spell the difference between success and failure of the program, not to mention the marriage. As time goes by it will not seem so trivial as it does now. If a husband and wife, or any other life partners, share the same aspiration and attitude toward healthful living, they have very considerable advantages right at the start. Not only will their health efforts profit by the harmony of their marriage (or partnership) but conversely their marriage (or partnership) will profit by the "hobby" they enjoy together.

If one partner is epicurean and hedonistic and derisively calls the other a "health nut," if one loves garlic and the other can't stand it, if one believes the low-fat diet propaganda and the other doesn't and enjoys a moderate amount of dietary fat, if one can't get along without meat and the other is a vegetarian, if one is frugal and the other wasteful, if one is religious and the other atheistic, we don't have to speculate on their chances of a harmonious marriage. It's not easy to be healthy when one's mate is a junky. It's just not true: Love does not solve all problems. "Love" is a siren song that should not be depended on too heavily. This is why the Bible admonishes, "Be not unequally yoked together."

As mundane as this matter may seem to be, I feel a couple contemplating marriage to each other should work for a clear understanding of the degree of commonality in their lives. If both partners enjoy organic gardening, for example, think how much they will enjoy nurturing their precious soil and earthworms together. No one will begrudge a late supper if both were out cultivating their garden together.

So, to persons who aspire to tie the knot of matrimony, put aside your rose-colored glasses for a spell and examine your relationship in the cold light of reality. With our marriages batting a sorry .670, or worse, we need all the harmony we can get.

Obviously, inherent compatibility alone is no assurance of a successful marriage. But not being a qualified counselor, I will not presume to teach you the fine points of marital success.

If you're not careful in selecting a wife, you may end up like this fellow who eventually discovered that to keep family harmony he always had to say, "Yes, ma'm. I'm sorry, ma'm. It'll never happen again."

Or consider this: There were two lines of men in a marriage counselor's waiting room. At the head of one line was a sign "For hen-pecked husbands." Three men were standing in it. The other line was labeled "For non-henpecked husbands." One man stood there. One of the henpecked men said to the fellow standing below the "non-henpecked" sign, "Hey, fella, you don't look like you belong there. You come stand here with us." The lonely one replied, "Well, I was going to stand in that line but my wife made me stand in this one."

One might well ask, "Which is more important for true health, a sound mind or a sound body?" I am tempted to say, "The mind is more important and the body is more important. But of course that's just my way of saying that it's futile to attempt to assign comparative merits to them. They are both essential parts of the whole, much as a husband and wife are both essential to their marriage.

We have all heard the term "psychosomatic," describing the mind's influence on the body. It has often been a convenient catch-all when the doctor is stymied by whatever is bothering the patient. But have you ever seen or heard the word "somatopsychotic?" Probably not, because I just now coined it not knowing whether it is an established term. But let's use it anyway to describe the body's effect on the mind which is given far less attention than it deserves.

Huge amounts of time, effort, and money are devoted to cure alcoholism, schizophrenia, nervous breakdowns other addictions, and all other forms of mental and personality maladies. But how many of these resources take into account the direct effect that body chemistry has on the mental processes, and consequently the personality of the patient? Blood sugar chemistry is often and indisputably implicated in mentally related cases. But far too many institutions, including the admirable and benevolent Alcoholics Anonymous, achieve what little success they do achieve, with mental strategies, will power, and other psychiatric approaches. Even psychiatry, that well entrenched and sophisticated science, seems to completely ignore the body-mind connection. Believe it or not. It's like fighting an unknown assailant, getting hit on the head and not knowing where the blows are coming from. Metabolically oriented researchers keep telling them and they keep ignoring the evidence. "Don't confuse me with the facts." I just can't help wondering: Is it because a five-year analysis is far more profitable than to actually cure (or to help Mother to cure)? A similar question applies to the slash, poison, and burn treatment for cancer. Is the $60,000 a factor?

We could not exist on this plane without a soul. And in turn a soul needs a mind. A mind needs a brain. A brain needs a body.

Does the quality of the brain depend on the quality of the body? I think we can say that for a certainty, because it is an integral part of the body, as we have said, and works interdependently and harmoniously with the rest of the body. Can we acknowledge then that if we want to live a quality life we unequivocally must have a quality body and that a quality body must have quality health?

Dr. Mortimer J. Adler, taking ideas from the "Great Books of the Western World," tells us that "physical fitness was held in high esteem in ancient Greece, the fountainhead of our intellectual culture... Thus the exercise of the body and of the mind went intimately together in ancient Athens and were pursued in the same place." Plato was a strong exponent of the body-mind relationship.

Dr. Adler tells us also that William James, the eminent physiologist, psychologist, and philosopher, was convinced that a "well-toned motor apparatus, nervous and muscular, was bound to have a wholesome effect on a person's state of mind and activity."

Scores of eminent authorities have expounded on the body's influence on the mind, thoughts, and actions. J. Edgar Hoover, former chief of the Federal Bureau of Investigation, emphasized that most of the crime in the U.S. was due to poor health caused by faulty diets. Dr. Deepak Chopra, author of the recent best-seller "Ageless Body, Timeless Mind," expresses the same opinion when he says, "I'm convinced from study that the root of crime today is poor health." He also says that the body-mind influence works both ways. When the endocrine system and nerves go awry senility results; the senility in turn inhibits the workings of the entire system. Dr. Chopra further says that a joyful person has a joyful body, light feet. A sad person has a sad body, heavy feet. A sick body produces a sick mind. The quality of mind determines the quality of awareness, and awareness is life itself. A healthy body is required for a truly worthy life.

Dr. Richard Horace Hoffman, psychiatrist, believed that "most neurotics are the way they are because some underlying and undiscovered bodily ailment contributes to their anxiety." He also felt that "the expression 'psychosomatic' was poorly chosen because so many people read into it a causative relation that was not originally intended. The notion that the mind causes somatic disease makes the tail wag the dog." I am in substantial accord with Dr. Hoffman on this.

Dr. E.M. Abrahamson, co-author of "Body, Mind and Sugar," says of the neurotic: "His brain is ill-nourished and tired from attempting to work without adequate fuel. ...Since the cells of the brain are those that depend wholly upon the moment-to-moment blood sugar level for nourishment, they are perhaps the most susceptible to damage. The large and ever-increasing number of neurotics in our population makes this clearly evident. ...We may say that these patients had suffered from hunger not only of the body but also of the mind. ...It now seems fairly obvious that low blood sugar...would be more likely to affect the nerve tissue adversely more than any other part of the body. ...Statistics show that low blood sugar is characteristic of schizophrenia. ...To do work adequately, whether it be mental, manual, or a combination of the two, requires a blood sugar level high enough to supply the normal demands of muscle, nerve, and brain cells. ...The brain, especially, needs sugar at all times."

While we're quoting, let's see what some others have to say on our subject.

"*A healthy body is a guest chamber for the soul; a sick body is a prison.*"
— Francis Bacon

"*To become a thoroughly good man is the best prescription for keeping a sound mind and a sound body.*"
— Francis Bowen

"*Age does not depend upon years, but upon the temperament and health. Some men are born old, and some never grow so.*"
— Tryon Edwards

"*A man is not old as long as he is seeking something.*"
— Jean Rostand

"*It must be of the spirit if we are to save the flesh.*"
— Douglas MacArthur

"*A cheerful heart is a good medicine, but a downcast spirit drieth up the bones.*"

— Proverbs 17:22

"*Most people would rather die than think; many do.*"

— Bertrand Russell

"*Closedmindedness is mental constipation, and you know how toxic constipation can be.*"

— Myself

As you can see, there are two sides to the coin of causation; some feel that the dog wags the tail and others feel that the tail wags the dog. More than a few feel that a considerable proportion of physical ills are generated by a sick mind. I think they are partly right. A sick mind will jeopardize one's well-being and interfere with the healing process, but I doubt that many illnesses are "caused" by mental instability. Exponents of this concept, I feel, are more philosophers than scientists; not saying that their philosophies are without merit.

Mental health is like money; it can't buy happiness but it certainly can keep you cheerful in your misery.

Many case histories on record show that sick people have regained their wholeness through their minds. Norman Cousins tells the world in his book, "*The Anatomy of An Illness*" that he overcame his cancer with a sense of humor. Purportedly he read and listened to numerous jokes, in other words laughing the malignancy out of his body. I don't doubt that he did do that. However, I still prefer to train my dog to wag his tail, because it's a much easier task than to try to train his tail to wag his body. I prefer to employ an approach that I can more easily understand and implement.

Physical measures taken to enhance my health are definitive and pragmatic and therefore more easily understood, whereas the mental, emotional, and spiritual approach is at best nebulous and does not present me anything to bite into. I could easily lose my resolve in such an endeavor. Positive thinking has its power but cannot be depended on to work. In fact, what determines the success or failure of positive thinking is the degree of success of whatever physical measures are taken to enhance health. If positive thinking inspires one to do something positive for his health, therein lies the power of positive thinking. While mental health does indeed tend to enhance physical health, my major message here is that because of the oneness of your whole being, physical health can go a long way in maintaining your general well-being and happiness. And the physical approach to health is simpler and easier. Though positive thinking can be a powerful adjunct to the physical approach, I will leave the power of positive thinking to someone else to contemplate.

This is a simple fact: If your body is impregnated with toxins, deficient in building blocks, lacking in tone and durability, and run-down from over-exertion and inadequate rest, brother, you're sick no matter how happy you are. A healthy mind and spirit make up only one-fifth of the five requisites for health I present here.

Your nervous system provides your body with its essential electrical energy without which your various parts will not function. This is not a figure of speech. Your nerve impulses are literally electrical impulses. In an experiment about 20 years ago electrodes were connected from a man's brain to a model electric train. With his thoughts alone the man moved, accelerated, and stopped the train. Keep your body clean, nourish it properly, keep it toned with enough exercise, give it enough rest to rejuvenate itself, and it will enable your nerves, including your brain, to power you to sparkling, energetic health.

If you question the interrelation and interdependence of the mind and body, observe a few feeble, doddering, unstable people. You'll notice that very few of them exhibit mental health. Their minds simply do not have a source of energy. If you place little importance in caring for your health, if you think it is not worth the effort, the day will surely come when you will change your mind.

Dr. Bruce Larson in his book "There's a Lot More to Health Then Not Being Sick" also shares many inspiring thoughts. Let's partake of them: Be hot or cold, not lukewarm. Be creative, taking sensible risks at times. To be always safe is dull and unhealthy. Your glands, physical and spiritual, stagnate with the sludge of boredom. Choose to live instead. Be alive all your life. Speak up and out. Contribute beneficially to society, even if it makes waves. Count for something. Don't be a walking dead. Lead your life; don't just ride along. Get into the front seat and drive, or pay for the ride, somehow. Don't let inertia bog you down. Every few years, change jobs and move geographically, if such a move would be advantageous. Have a project going or planned. Look forward to the future. Life is not a destination but a continuing journey. Your life doesn't have to be an extension of your past and present, unless it's already on an upward bias. If life isn't treating you right, change it to suit yourself. Whatever the mind can conceive, the mind and body can do. So step out in faith, and that faith will soon grow and provide the power for your project, because a worthy cause will release the power to accomplish it.

Make a hobby of health. Have a purpose of life. What better medium can one have than working toward perfection of the temple of the Holy Spirit? Learning new ways that succeed will continuously encourage you and give you fresh enjoyment of life. You will remain vibrant and vigorous all your life and will die young at an old age.

Brothers and sisters, to succeed in your pursuit of health you must know who and what will help you and who and what will work against you. Just for a moment, free yourself from the yoke of faith you have in the Unholy Trinity, if you do have such faith, a yoke you desperately carry for lack of knowledge. Listen to and read what these moneyed industrialists say and write, observe what they do, and appraise their results. Now connect all the dots and you will see a picture develop. Well, lo and behold! The picture is a dollar sign! Is your faith appropriately placed?

We all are responsible for our own health, whether we acknowledge it or not. Go ahead and blame it on your doctor. Or blame your tribulations on chance. It doesn't matter. If you're sick, you're sick. Let's stop regarding cancer as though it were a number which popped up in a lottery. Cancer, like everything else, is very much subject to the laws of cause and effect. If you attract it consistently enough it will accommodate you. Live by Mother's laws and you need not be the one-in-three who will succumb to the Big C. (Statistics now are reportedly fast approaching one-in-two.) Is this admonishment just a bunch of hassle to you, a killjoy, a wet blanket? A thirty-three percent chance says you could some day regret your reliance on your sixty-seven percent chance of avoiding the scourge. The probability of your succumbing to the Big C is approaching fifty percent.

If you really want to know what health is about and how to care for it, seek the guidance of the One who created you and your body. Then listen. You could learn a lot. How do I know? I consult with Him very often, and He has spoken to my spirit. My spirit in turn has searched and learned, guiding me in my study and experiments.

> *"If a million people say a stupid thing, it is still a stupid thing."*
>
> — T.C. Fry

> *"If a dog has four legs and you consider his tail to be a leg, how many legs does he have? He still has only four legs."*
>
> — Abraham Lincoln

Let's not seek false security by sticking with the crowd. You may find comfort in knowing you are not alone in your erratic thinking, and if you also find comfort in knowing that a million others are also sick along with you, be consoled that millions of others also find the same comfort. But if you're sick, you're sick. Be that as it may.

Remember this: Education alone does not make a good doctor. Bad education is worse than no education. But worse yet is the doctor's attitude toward his profession and how he practices it. Big Medi$in has fostered many superstitions in its patients. We assume we're healthy until some outside factor, like germs or the weather, attacks us. We have no control over what befalls us, even though we're supposed to be the smartest entities on earth. On the other hand, the more "primitive" people at least know that one's illness is a result of one's wrongdoing. It's not mere loose talk when I say that America's medical "knowledge" is fraught with more damaging superstitions than that of the witch doctor.

Lord Woolsey said of the King of England: "Be careful what you put into his head, because you'll never get it out again." Don't you be like the king. There's abundant good information out here to replace what you "know" — and to your benefit. Joseph Addison said, "Reading is to the mind what exercise is to the body." To this I might add that books are your exercise equipment and your library is the gymnasium for your mind.

Just for a laugh let's look at a few superstitions:

"The world is flat."

"Bleeding is good therapy." It is said that George Washington was bled to death in an attempt to cure a sore throat.

"We can restore and maintain health by poisoning the body." This is a big superstition in vogue today. Like the former two, it will eventually come in for its share of justified ridicule. But you'd better not wait for that day, because if you do, that hocus pocus will kill you before your time. The only way to be healthy is to maintain conditions in your body conducive to health, and that does not include poisoning.

Such huge amounts of time, effort, and money are spent on remedies for the thriving illnesses of America. Whatever has become of the old adage that an ounce of prevention is worth a pound of cure? It doesn't seem to be an exaggeration to say that for every ton of "remedy" in orthodox medicine there's hardly an ounce of prevention. After all, disease is just a matter of chance. This is America, land of the free. But what good is this brand of freedom if it breeds catastrophic conditions throughout the land? The free enterprise system is a great ideal but we just can't live on ideals. But what I think doesn't matter. Big Medi$in isn't going to back down for me. So there's only one solution for me if I want to be healthy, and that is to achieve and maintain my own health. Unfortunately, or fortunately, the same applies to you.

Good habits are not just a trivial subject preached to you by your sixth grade hygiene teacher. They are an essential part of your successful health regimen, as well as your successful life in general. Do a thing a second time and it begins to be a habit, good or bad. If it's a good one, feed it along with repetitions. If it's a bad one, knock it off — right now. Remember, if you stop a good habit, you're starting a bad one, or at least a less-than-ideal condition.

I realize that probably a huge percentage of health seekers give up in frustration. Eventually they say, "Oh, what's the use?" and give up their ambitions for a long and vigorous life. If you're one of these souls, I'm here to tell you that I understand and that it's not hard to be healthy. First I strongly suggest that you return to the chapter on internal cleanliness and reread the discussions on amalgam dental fillings, root canals, and intestinal flora. These three factors can be serious and unrecognized deterrents to health. They are insidious in undermining one's health. Because of them probably millions have gone through years of wondering why they are always sub-par no matter how hard they try to be healthy. I would say it would behoove everyone to explore these possibilities. There may be other similar mysterious deterrents to health I don't know about. You might explore these possibilities if you haven't found a solution to your health problems.

Another deterrent to success in health is lack of patience. Don't be like the impatient vulture who was anxious to kill something. You must allow a few months for results to show. In the meantime, maintain your faith in your program. Realize that nothing but good can come out of your efforts.

311

You are making up for a deficit in your health condition, and when you have filled that hole you will begin to see the results pile up. If you persevere you will be rewarded. I speak from experience, once being a miserable, puny wretch. I had most of the classic chronic ailments, being old far before my time. Now I have no chronic ailments to speak of.

About a year ago I had a heartening experience. My wife and I visited an orthopedist for a shoulder injury I acquired in a fall on ice. As we examined the x-rays my wife said, "Oh what cute little bones you have!" The doctor said, "I'm not looking at his bones. Everybody's bones look the same. I'm looking at the spaces between the bones. Notice how clean they are. This man has no arthritis." Now, let me tell you, I once had arthritis, or bursitis, for many years in both shoulders. Only after I quit following the Pied Piper and started on the straight and narrow did I free myself of my many ills. I promise you, you can be healthy too, to whatever degree your efforts warrant.

I once opened a fortune cookie and was pleased to read, "In nature there are no rewards and no punishments — only consequences." That's karma, isn't it? And it's true, and that's what is so great about this life of ours. So paddle your canoe with the knowledge that you have a brother here who understands and is pulling for you too.

"*There is no dependence that can be sure but a dependence upon one's self.*"

— John Gay

"*As long as a man does and thinks only as he is told, he is a slave. The moment he thinks for himself, he is a free man.*"

— Anonymous

"Experience is not what happens to you; it is what you do with what happens to you."

— Aldous Huxley

"The quality of life depends largely on the liver." How's that for a neat little double entendre?

It is true that your liver is one very important organ. It has been described as having more than 500 functions in the service of your body. It participates in a major way in the processing of food and building your blood while also being a major cleaner-upper. As long as your liver is functioning as intended you're at least in pretty good health. Where cancer has set in, we know that the liver has lost its efficiency and has failed to maintain health. So love your liver and treat it fairly. Learn more about it and keep it healthy.

Now, what about the other liver referred to above? You. Yes, the quality of your life depends very heavily on you and what you do with your life. A truly quality life comprises a quality body, including the brain, a quality mind, and a quality spirit. In other words, you simply must be a good man, a good woman, or a good child. And incidentally, a quality life automatically includes happiness; and isn't happiness, after all, what it's all about?

You're basically okay, made in the image of God. So be yourself, as free as you can be from all the adverse and distracting influences to which we humans fall prey. Most of us learned how to do this in early childhood but got pulled off the straight and narrow by the trials of life. That's very natural and to be expected, but there's no law that says we should let life buffet us around and determine for us how we live. I don't have to tell you about such traits as honesty, sincerity, industriousness, compassion, perseverance, love, faith,

313

patience, responsibility, gratitude, and all the other traits that go to make a quality person. But I would like to inspire you to realize and duly appreciate the validity and advantages of living on a high plane.

Be your own person and don't get sucked in by Madison Avenue, and you know that Big Medi$in is one of the pillars of Madison Avenue. And if you really are your own, you're always in charge of your affairs, not your doctor. If you will study a bit, you will know more practical facts about your body than your doctor will. Never again say, "You're the doctor; you know best." You don't have to be part of the statistics that say "one out of three will get cancer." Given half-a-chance your body will stand strong and not succumb.

The most successful people, the happiest people, are those who are a bit different, who do things a bit differently, and a bit better than the crowd. So give up trying to fit into the mold designed and dictated by others. Create your own unique mold. Be free and healthy in mind and body.

Let's stop being confused in our perception of the cause and effect of disease. Let's untwist our minds. We are not victims of disease; we are the cause of it. We can control it if we will. We need to thoroughly know this and always remember it. The task before us, the action which will enhance and glorify our lives, is to exercise our abilities and responsibilities.

People who summarily reject new ideas do so for at least two reasons: (1) They are free riders who choose not to participate in the building of our world, allowing others to do the work or (2) they regard their own intellects and philosophies as being inferior and not worthy of contributing to our pool of knowledge. They are the type who depend on the architect to decide for them how they are to live in their home. Don't you be one of these. Be the important person that you are.

Granted, the desire for social approval is the second-strongest instinct in man. But that doesn't mean you must have it. All it means is that normal human beings find comfort in knowing that others respect them. You can rise above the norm. If you have enough self respect you won't have a crying need for the respect or even approval of others. And self respect comes from being willing to stand up for what's right and against the fallacies of society. Obey the laws. Love the earth and its creatures. This probably sounds corny to those who haven't freed themselves from the second-strongest instinct. It requires maturity.

Honesty promotes tranquillity of soul. Dishonesty keeps the mind, conscious and subconscious, on edge and stressed, and we know that stresses are one of the sources of free radicals, and also that the major ambition of free radicals is to age us before our time.

Do we find discomfort in being called a "health nut?" Not I. You may call me that any time. In fact that term is gaining more respect every day, now that more people are wising up to the fallacy of the medical status quo. "Health nut" is a badge of intelligence and responsibility. Cherish it. I do.

As intelligent and responsible health nuts we should recognize the subtle danger of getting to accept, even love, the flavors of commonly used synthetic chemicals. Understandably, so many people routinely drink perfumey beverages and love the flavors. I admit to still enjoying the lovely synthetic flavoring in strawberry soda water. I'll bet you do too. Oh, well...

"I never make predictions, especially about the future."

— Yogi Berra

This little cutie from Yogi is not meant to have anything to do with anything. I just thought you needed a respite from my preaching. To be truly healthy we need humility, and that means we need to see ourselves as we truly are. As human beings we all have inherent limitations and room for improvement. This improvement can be achieved by receiving help from others, either other people or perhaps a higher power. But some people are reluctant to seek help from others, because they feel that seeking outside help is a sign of weakness and lack of confidence. Nothing could be further from the truth, for it really is a sign of strength, self-confidence, and humility, as well as a means of acquiring strength and wisdom in excess of what one possesses on his own. It takes strength and courage to acknowledge one's own limitations. If one appreciates the blessings bestowed on him by his Creator and maintains a partnership with Him, he possesses a confidence and strength which gives him a special advantage in the affairs of his life.

Similarly, it takes strength and courage to acknowledge one's ignorance, even though ignorance is merely not knowing something, and we know that nobody knows everything. Those who refuse to acknowledge their own normal ignorance tend to remain ignorant. Admitting ignorance and lack of wisdom will free you from the shackles of false pride and allow you to seek knowledge and wisdom and thereby enhance your stature as a person. And isn't that one of the major goals we should be striving for?

A few more thoughts to reflect on the body-mind relationship:

We are what we eat and what we think.
To think is to practice brain chemistry.
Love produces good chemistry and enhances health.
Laughter makes healing chemistry.
Spirit is the silent spaces between thoughts.
Intuition is cell chemistry.
Good thoughts can produce anti-cancer chemicals.
Anger produces destructive chemicals.
Depression speaks to every cell in the body and is carcinogenic.
Closed-mindedness is mental constipation.

Let's close this section by observing how a mentally healthy person resolves problems and frustrations:

1. He tries to remedy the situation.

2. If remedy is not achieved, he tries to relieve himself by giving vent to his emotions by speaking with someone about the frustration. Or he may blow his steam by expressing his emotions with some physical activity.

3. If the problem is still unresolved, he may choose to accept the status quo.

4. If he cannot accept the status quo, he may leave the field, divorcing himself from the scene altogether.

EXERCISE

I know you're smart enough to know this, and I don't want to speak down to you, but the rules of literary safety dictate that I say it, lest some bleeding-heart medical entity jump on me for practicing medicine without a license. So:

If you have any doubts about your physical condition, especially if you're elderly or feeble, consult with your physician before starting any physical exercise.

Exercise, physical and mental, enhances circulation, health, and life. Sloth is stagnation and is in the direction of disease, nothingness, and death. But, as in almost all other aspects of life, there is a choice. But this choice is not optional; it is mandatory. The privilege of choice is not a free lunch; it is an onus placed on us as the price we pay for the privilege of having the choice. We also may choose to do it intentionally or unintentionally; voluntarily or by default. If we do not choose to exercise, by default we choose not to exercise.

Inertia can be a friend or foe, depending on how we choose. In either case it will fortify the results of our choice. If we choose to exercise, inertia will reward us by making the activity pleasurable or at least gratifying. If we choose, voluntarily or not, not to exercise, inertia will accommodate us with further slothfulness.

"Movers and shakers" is a phrase applied to people of account, people who live and help others to live. So if you would really live and make your short stay on earth a worthy one, move and shake — in body, mind, and soul.

> "*Dost thou love life? Then do not squander time, for that is the stuff life is made of.*"
>
> — Benjamin Franklin

> "*Even if you're on the right track, you'll get run over if you just sit there.*"
>
> — Arthur Godfrey

For us ordinary people the primary objective in physical exercise should not be only to build powerful muscles but, more importantly, to tone all the components of the body so that, like the instruments of a fine musical orchestra, they may play sweet music in harmony with one another. This objective of course does not necessarily apply to certain individuals who, for money, personal glory, or other reasons, need or desire a powerful body in order to succeed at what they aspire to.

Exercise doesn't have to be strenuous to help. In fact, on a per-effort basis the greatest benefit comes at the start of exercise. The breakout of stagnation is a quantum leap. The difference in well-being is greater between stagnation and moderate exercise than between moderate and heavy exercise. Heavier exercise, within limits, of course may be more beneficial than moderate, especially because of the aerobics involved, but the major benefits have already been accrued from just overcoming inertia by stimulating the metabolism.

Strenuous exercise is not quite "normal" for most of us these days and so can sometimes yield adverse results. If it is not continued as a lifestyle, its aftermath can be somewhat less than salubrious, if not detrimental and hazardous. Observe the following few examples.

When World War II broke out, many forms of public entertainment were curtailed. The professional flyweight champion fighter of Hawaii, whose weight class was 112 pounds and under, ballooned out to 175 pounds before the war was over. Few people realize how strenuous fight training is.

Some years ago I read that the average life span of professional athletes was 55 years. Soon after that, Jackie Robinson died at age 53. You may recall that he was the first black baseball player to be admitted into the major leagues. Before that he played baseball, football, and other sports at the University of California at Los Angeles. I don't know whether 55 is really the average life span of professional athletes, but the coincidence intrigued me.

Buster Douglas, who weighed about 250 pounds when he took the heavyweight boxing title from Mike Tyson a

319

few years ago, weighed 400 pounds recently. I'm not optimistic about Buster's future and hope he doesn't add credibility to the 55-year average.

One day a chubby young lady came into our body-toning salon to inquire about our services. She and her husband had been running about five miles every day for several months and had felt pretty healthy. But then he broke his arm at work and they both stopped running. She told me he gained 25 pounds in the couple months since and that she gained 20. As she appeared to be in her twenties, I presume, or hope, that they both eventually regained at least a modicum of physical well-being.

Even though nobody else seems concerned about this yo-yo practice of off-and-on strenuous physical exertion, I'm sticking with my concern over it, because it's logical and I've seen many results of the practice. Now, I'm not saying that nobody should go into strenuous sports, because numerous people have gloriously enhanced their lives through sports, and the price is well worth paying. Quid pro quo again.

Let me round out this discussion of the hazards of hot-and cold exertion with two hypothetical stories:

John, young and in good health with clean coronary arteries, gets into a heavy running regimen, doing about eight miles every other day. After six months he quits running. He probably will suffer no serious adverse results, though he may gain a few unwelcome pounds.

But let's say Pete, age 46, is diagnosed by his cardiologist as being pretty clogged up in his coronary arteries and advised to get into an adequately aerobic activity. So he begins a running program and soon gets to enjoy it. He gradually builds up his endurance and after eight months is running eight miles every other day. He's feeling much healthier now, because his blocked arteries have enlarged some and numerous new capillaries have developed to accommodate the new demands of the new physical activity. To his dismay Pete is sent on a working trip by his employer, the duration thereof being undetermined. His mission is demanding, requires long hours of stressful work, and leaves no time for running, as heavy time demands are imposed by the customer. The quality of his diet "on the road" deteriorates, consisting mostly of hamburgers, hot dogs, fries, and soft drinks — whenever he can find time for them. Two months into the trip Pete falls victim to a heart attack.

How in the world! Wasn't Pete supposed to be in good shape? Yes, as long as he was running. But he began to go downhill shortly after he stopped running. But why so soon? Before he started running he was in no real danger; so why should he have any worries now, even after eight months of running? Consider the following:

It is said that a month after stopping a serious exercise program a person has lost about 80 percent of his "training effect."

The original blockage in Pete's arteries was probably due to less-than-ideal living habits. Since he felt pretty good while running, he probably didn't bother to improve his diet. The increased blood supply to his heart gave him a new sense of well-being. In fact he was healthier — for the time being. So what happened to Pete to bring on his troubles? Here's what I think: His new capillaries, now relieved of their challenge, shrank back to almost nothing and his arteries shrank back to original size. So far it seems he should be back to square one. But he's not; he's further back, somewhere behind the eight-ball. For the sake of a happy ending, let's say that Pete survived the attack fairly well; he didn't die.

At least two conditions did Pete in. First, while his arteries were larger and made him complacent, unbeknown to him more cholesterol was being deposited on the walls of his arteries, largely through his sticking with the standard American diet, also known as SAD. Still it was okay as long as the vessels remained open and spacious. But when the running stopped and the arteries contracted to their original size, their inside diameter, including the new deposits of cholesterol, was now smaller than before, decreasing the rate of blood flow and increasing the pressure. But that's not all; since Pete quit running he added eight pounds to his already overloaded frame, imposing an additional burden on his poor heart. The attack is not at all surprising. Can you see why I feel any heavy exercise program should be approached with caution and good judgment?

Now, what about John, the fellow who suffered no serious effects of his abrupt cessation of strenuous running? First, he was in good shape to begin with; in other words he had a good cushion to fall on, adequate inside diameter to his arteries for the free flow of blood. But had he been older and obese, he might have also put himself in danger. He got away this time but he had better not be so cavalier about his health in the future, especially as he grows older and puts on more weight.

Most competitive sports are not necessarily the type of exercise we should associate with the pursuit of health. The health benefits they offer are only incidental to other benefits, such as self esteem, social adulation, and financial gain. Further, they are not easily regulated to produce optimum health benefits. In fact, demands made on the body by competition are sometimes inimical to health, not to mention the severe injuries occasioned by the rigors of competition.

"Physical fitness" is not synonymous with health. Recall the case of Jim Fixx, a leading advocate and exponent of heavy running, who died of a heart attack while running. On the other hand, look at the late Paul Bragg, health guru to movie stars. He was not a competitive athlete but he was healthy. At age 78 he swam the English Channel and at 79 climbed the Matterhorn. I ran with him on the sands of Waikiki when he was 78 and was amazed at the man's extraordinary physical conditioning.

All things considered, the exercise I like best is that which is part of everyday living. We should make the most of our daily chores and supplement them with other exercise as warranted. A profitable attitude is to duly appreciate the physical actions necessitated by a wholesome and productive life. Try to shun labor-saving devices. When massaging yourself or another, favor the use of your hands over an electric vibrator. The electrical energy from the vibrator is no match for the living energy from loving hands. Give away, or at least limit the use of, your electric roast slicer, food processor, cake mixer, tooth brush, razor, leaf blower, and other such calorie savers. If you're physically up to it, till your garden with hand tools rather than a power tiller. The trick in all this is to consciously enjoy the physical effort involved. Notice that I said to <u>consciously</u> enjoy it. Thus your exuberant emotional state will activate the metabolic processes salubrious to your mind and body.

If you can attain this healthy attitude you will not bemoan having to walk back to the tool shed to get your shovel. Instead you will happily stride back with a resolute spirit and pep in your step and hustle in your muscle, realizing that blessed is he who can walk and work. My senior neighbor has told me more than once, "Oh how I wish I could work like you."

The only additional exercise you will need is that which will raise your pulse and breathing to a level where you feel healthfully stimulated. The conventional wisdom is to do this for 20 or 30 minutes three or four times a week. Any more than that will garner you less and less benefit per unit of energy spent.

The discussion on exercise immediately above was simplified and generalized. You should consult some of the excellent books available on the subject. But a standard for the optimal degree of exertion in health exercise has been accepted as being about 75 percent of your maximum pulse (heartbeats per minute). Your maximum pulse is 220 minus your age. For example, if you're 30 years old your maximum pulse is 220 minus 30, or 190. Your optimum pulse is 75 percent of 190, or 143. If you're 55 the pulse you should maintain for 20 to 30 minutes is 75 percent of (220 minus 55), or 124. Much more than this will not yield much better results. Remember that Socrates said, "Be moderate in all things." Need I remind you that you should work up to these standards of exertion slowly?

A person in his twilight years should resolve to maintain an active life. If he has a single-family home and yard to care for, this can be a great boon to him. A person living in a rented apartment, or the like, has a real challenge before him. Isn't it a pity that so many retirees opt for the rocking chair instead of the spading fork? An elderly person's exercise should be at least the equivalent of walking a mile every day or two miles every other day. He should resolve to shun the siren song of the rocking chair or sofa except for an occasional respite during an active day or as a well deserved rest and digestion of the benefits of his day of healthful activity. The older a person is, the more he needs and benefits from exercise.

The state of health of today's average person has come to be accepted as "standard" or "normal." That's unfortunate, because it has resulted in shortened lives of poorer quality. Sickness in old age has become the norm, inevitably occurring when the whole body has given up after years of stalwart service fighting the abuse by its owner. It's all too easy to accept the status quo, because everybody else does, and it's comfy to do as everybody else does. After all, mediocrity, while nothing to brag about, is still good enough to keep one in the ballpark.

I'm here to tell you there is a better way. It takes effort, but the first wall of resistance is the toughest, and once you've knocked it over, the remaining ones will be easier, and you will be exhilarated and proud of having had the gumption to be willing to pay for something of value. It has been solidly determined after extensive study and experience over the breadth of our land and decades of time, that physical exercise is a decided requisite for true health.

Let us look at how exercise enhances our well-being:

(1) Exercise enhances all metabolic functions: organs and glands, circulation of nutritive and cleansing factors (blood and lymph), pulmonary capacity, heart strength and durability, excretory functions (bowels, skin, lungs, and urinary system), the mind (product of the physical brain), bones; in short, health.

(2) Muscular strength is essential to good health. It goes together with strength of our inner workings. Remember that all our body parts are intimately interdependent on one another. A person with hanging flab not only lacks the ability to push or lift a heavy load; his whole physiology

325

is weak and vulnerable to any and all adversity which may come along. Body functions are in stagnation. Endurance is lacking. It has been said that the tissues of flabby people are rancid and in a state of decay. Remember that rancidity is a major carcinogen. This is not a happy thought but sadly it may be true.

(3) Exercise tones the nerves, which in turn maintain a healthy mental and emotional state, which returns the favor by helping to maintain a good physical tone. This is a symbiotic, or even a synergistic, relationship.

(4) Exercise, especially when your juices are happily flowing, is like the flow of a lively stream; refreshing, nourishing, and cleansing.

(5) Exercise prolongs the prime of life. Let's do some practical hypothesizing. Percy is 30 and realizes that his way of life is predisposing him to a premature attrition of his health and a shortening of his life. After some study and contemplation he decides to do moderately aerobic exercise for 30 minutes three times a week for the rest of his life. He perseveres and lives to 80. Let's just say he would have died at 75 had he lived a sedentary life. Over the 50 years Percy put in 3900 hours of exercise. The five years of extended life he gained through his exercise program amounted to 43,800 hours. So in Percy's case each hour of exercise netted him 11.2 hours of extra life. He also earned a dividend of 50 years of fairly vigorous health instead of 45 years of a mediocre and "normal" life, complete with the occasional incidence of illness which goes with the territory. If we can say that our assumptions of how Percy's life turned out were not unreasonably optimistic, then we can say that Percy worked out a pretty good deal for himself. Further assuming that a person who exercises seriously probably also observes a judicious diet and shuns tobacco, alcohol,

and other vices, we can readily see the considerable benefits that come with a conscientious and responsible lifestyle.

Have you noticed how some people begin to walk and move like old folks when they get to be about 50? Don't you be like them. Exercise. Use your mind and spirit to help you keep young. Someone has said, "It's not so much that old men sit around. It's more that when men sit around they grow old."

On the average, statistically, blue-collar workers outlive white-collar workers and are healthier to boot.

But we know that a conscientious and responsible lifestyle is more easily discussed than done. Making changes, especially substantial and meaningful ones, is usually difficult. But we also know that worthwhile results seldom come easy. We must bear down with a healthy dose of resolve to follow through. Remember what we were taught as youngsters, that "perseverance conquers all"?

Ironically, when we're feeling slothful and absolutely don't feel like exercising, that's when we need it most. I've said this to myself many times, and it's got me off my derriere many times. It's a great statement to commit to memory. So I've made a pronounceable acronym of it and posted it on my wall. Perhaps you would like to do the same. Here it is: WIDFLE, TWINIM, "When I don't feel like exercising, that's when I need it most." When I don't have the strength to overcome the heavy stagnation of my inner and outer machinery, I look at WIDFLE, TWINIM and say, "Well, I guess I gotta do a little at least, so I'll know I haven't reneged on my program and myself. Besides, a little exercise is better than none." So I reluctantly jump up and do it. Almost every time, once I overcome the initial resistance, my inners produce and circulate the juices that stimulate my enthusiasm and fuel my continued exercise. I also remind

327

myself that missing a scheduled exercise session is already the start of terminating the program and letting myself down. I also gain strength through prayer. Should I nevertheless fail to keep an appointment with myself, I make a stronger effort not to miss a second one, for I know that a repeated act is a formation of a habit, bad or good, and that a second miss is exponentially more powerful than the first in leading me in the wrong direction. If I miss a third successive appointment, I've put myself at a very great disadvantage and must assume the difficult task of getting myself back on track. This failure probably happens to most of us, but we just have to stand up against it if we aspire to enrich our lives with good health.

Conversely, the more times we meet our schedule without missing, the stronger our good habit becomes and the more likely will be the success of our program. Another good idea is to make our exercise enjoyable, if not fun. But be sure that your fun activity also provides the required aerobic stimulation. Having a partner of like aspirations also helps, especially if commitments are made to each other.

Incidentally, I may as well tell you of a few acronyms I've added to WIDFLE, TWINIM: YAGBYEWHAP, "Ya ain't gonna build your endurance without huffing and puffing." YAGSABAL, "Ya also gotta sweat and burn a little." INAWOT, "It's not a waste of time." IWEM, "It's worth every minute." EMYR, "Every minute yields results." These acronyms have been extremely valuable to me, because I enjoy sitting and watching TV as much as most people.

Enough theory. Let's get moving. Here I'm going to describe one of my favorite sets of exercises. They are a good adjunct to a reasonably active lifestyle. Though not very aerobic, they will do a lot to preserve your youth, because by doing them you will "open up" and loosen the parts of your body, shaking out the stagnation which prevailed while you were at rest. You should appreciate hearing the many little "clicks" in your body that will signal to you that you are now a mover and shaker. The exercises are easy to do and, depending on your attitude, probably enjoyable. They are done in bed, before you get up to greet the rest of your day. They can take five minutes or however long you care to enjoy them. Thus they have a high degree of sustainability. What I say here is just a rough guide. Improvise and innovate for yourself, because benefits are more easily obtained from exercises you do with gusto. Moreover, these exercises can easily be modified and adapted for use anytime in the course of your day when you're up and around.

I hope you will do these the rest of your life, in one form or another. I call these exercises: Stretch, Bend, Twist, Flex, and Breathe.

You may want to go to the bathroom before getting into the routine. If you do, get back into bed for the exercises. Two general rules: (1) Hold every extended position for a few seconds, for the following reasons: (a) Your cells, your tissues, your nerves require time to relax and adjust to the new position. (b) Your lubricating juices (synovial fluid) require time to enter the spaces opened up for them. I don't have to tell you that the healthier you have kept yourself, the better will be the quality of the fluid which will cleanse, lubricate, and nourish your joints. (2) Whenever a move causes a slight pain (a "catch," a twinge, a "pull"), try to work the pain out by gently working through it, left and right, back and forth. The instructions below may look somewhat detailed on paper but will be simpler once you get started. So let's get started.

STRETCH. Lying on your back, elongate your body as much as you can. Bring your lumbar area down into contact with the bed surface, by tilting your pelvis upward. Extend your arms upward, toward the head of the bed, bending your elbows if the headboard or wall is in your way. Now stretch your whole self and feel all your joints open up and other tissues extend as well. Include your fingers and toes in the fun. Ideally, all of the following exercises involve stretching also. As you bend, twist, flex, and breathe, think "stretch."

LONG SIDE BENDS. Lying on your back with legs extended, move head and both feet to one side. Reach down with your hand and touch your knee on the same side. Consciously feel and relish the stretch in the other side of your whole body. Repeat in the other direction.

SHORT SIDE BENDS. Lying on your back with knees drawn up, repeat what you did in the Long Side Bends, immediately above. Bend enough that you can see and touch your feet as you bend. Again, consciously feel the pull on the other side. Repeat in the other direction.

LONG FRONT BEND. Lying on your back with legs extended, raise your feet and head simultaneously. Be moderate here, as you could easily strain the tendons in the backs of your legs. This bend offers much benefit to your lower back as well as your abdominal muscles.

SHORT FRONT BEND. Lying on your back, bring both knees up and hold them there with your hands. Bend your head forward and try to touch your chin to your knees, both knees together, then each knee alternately. While pulled up, you might massage your back a bit by rolling side-to-side and rocking backward and forward.

BACK BEND. From lying on your back, turn to one side and reach your hands, head, and feet backwards, forming an arch from your hands to your feet. Don't hesitate to twist around a bit to distribute the benefits to more joints and tissues. Repeat in the other direction.

LONG TWIST. Lying on your back with legs extended, bring one foot over the other and reach with it as far as you comfortably can to the other side. Turn your head in the direction opposite the reaching foot. You will feel a good pull in your joints and tissues but you can increase the benefit by consciously rotating your pelvic structure in the direction of the reaching foot. Now, that's what you call a twist. Repeat in the other direction. Do not wax too enthusiastic on this one, as you could easily overstress something. This is why I ask you to consciously feel your movements.

SHORT TWIST. Lying on your back with knees drawn up, repeat what you did in the Long Twist described above. Notice a little different effect. Remember to twist your pelvic structure.

FLEX. Flex as many muscles as you can throughout your whole body. Innovate your own moves. For example, with your hands around your knees, you can pull yourself up into a tight little ball and with your muscles try to squeeze yourself even smaller. You can also press hard against the mattress with both arms as if trying to lift your body off the mattress, simultaneously pointing your feet. Flex so you can feel the effects in your calves, quadriceps (fronts of your thighs), buttocks, and triceps, as well as the muscles of your torso. Bend your toes down hard as if trying to clench a fist with your feet. Bend them up also. Squeeze hard with your hands to make tight fists.

A special note on HANDS AND FEET. What you did for your main body you can generally do for your hands and feet. Stretch, bend, twist, and flex them, as well as every

331

finger and toe separately. Your feet need the help of your hands but your hands can do each other very well. With a little imagination and initiative, you can do a surprising number of things with, to, and for your hands. I would be remiss if I failed to mention that your hands and feet contain many reflex points that impinge on the well-being of your entire body. These points may be called acupuncture or acupressure points. Reflexology will be discussed soon.

BREATHE. For many years I regarded deep breathing a somewhat wimpish exercise, thinking that its effects were nebulous and not dynamic enough to be bothered with. Not anymore. It helped me immeasurably a few years ago in Mexico when I suffered severe allergic congestion in my head and lungs from Guadalajara's allergenic climate. I will never belittle deep breathing again.

Specialists on the subject often, if not always, differentiate between chest breathing and "stomach" breathing, saying that stomach (diaphragm, really) breathing is the proper way to breathe. The art of breathing is very much part of the wisdom of the Far East and an essential part of the Yoga discipline. So you may want to explore the literature on the subject.

In addition to the matter of stomach breathing I have some well considered thoughts on the whys and hows of breathing. First, remember that oxygen is the most essential element to almost all life, especially man's. The more air we take in, the more oxygen we deliver to our cells. The more we expand the air cells of the sponge which is our lungs, the more effective will be our lungs and the more alive will be our entire body. The more thoroughly we empty our lungs with each exhalation, the more impurities will be unloaded from our system and the more air and oxygen will we be able to take in with the next inhalation. The more regularly and habitually we maximize the expansion and compression of our lungs, the more regularly and thoroughly will we fulfill the function of our breathing. And cumulatively that's a lot of breathing.

Over and above supplying oxygen to our cells and unloading impurities through our lungs, correct deep breathing can do an effective job of expelling congestive mucus from our head and lungs. Such a need arises when we are beset with a cold or allergic attack. I learned this first-hand in a pleasantly surprising experience, which I mentioned just a few lines above. I was in Guadalajara, Mexico, and contemplating returning home to escape a very disabling allergic reaction to Guadalajara's allergenic atmosphere. My lungs were so loaded with mucus (more specifically called "phlegm" when in the lungs) that I involuntarily played all kinds of musical melodies with each exhalation. The misery was so great as to induce me to try anything I could think of to relieve my discomfort and restore at least a modicum of comfort until I got out of there. As so often happens in times of desperation, I resorted to theorizing on how best to get the bothersome material out of my lungs. I thought of my lungs as being two sponges, and to myself I said, "A sponge is more effectively cleaned out if filled completely and then completely squeezed with a forceful impetus." So I began to inhale more deeply than usual and exhale faster and with more force than usual. At first I noticed no response other than the music I already had been playing. But I persevered anyway. After more than several additional repetitions, lo and behold, something seemed to be happening in there. I was encouraged to further persevere, and after a few more minutes my efforts rewarded me with a small amount of mucus which came up with surprising ease. What a surprise!

In the next few minutes I got a little bit more of the stuff out but not much. However, I noticed that breathing was definitely a bit easier and less music was produced. So I continued the special breathing, remembering to inhale through the nose and exhale through the mouth. After another few minutes I decided to take a breather (pun intended) and come back to this encouraging exercise a bit later on.

As I sat at my typewriter in the process of writing this book I was spontaneously surprised again. Just in the course of normal breathing another bit of viscous fluid came up, and without any effort on my part. "Golly, what in the world is happening here?" I concluded that the forceful compression of my lungs had squeezed some of the extraneous material out of the lungs and into the bronchial area where it was no longer trapped in the cells of the lungs. It was now sitting free enough to be lifted up and out by the force of normal exhalation. What's more, this involuntary action was repeated occasionally during the course of the day.

A similar thing was happening in my nasal passages. Now I understand why "they" always advocate inhaling through the nose and exhaling through the mouth: With the inhaled air streaming through the nasal passages, whatever is in there is carried along with the air into the throat area, where it is now in position for expulsion. Exhalation through the mouth ensures that it is carried in the right direction.

Not resting on these fortuitous happenings, I continued to pursue my special breathing exercises. And the rewards kept coming. My breathing got closer and closer to being silent and normal and in a few days was back to normal.

The down side of this episode of relief was that without a radio with me I had to live without music.

If you do these exercises when you have a chest cold or any other congestion in your chest, you may expect to experience involuntary coughs. This is part of the purging process and will hasten your recovery and diminish as your lungs clear up.

As related earlier, I also resorted to a green vegetable juice fast when the allergy affected me. And so I can't say for a certainty which was the more effective remedy, the green drink fast or the deep breathing exercise. But I think I can safely say that the green drink did its job chemically and the breathing did its job by physical means. Anyway my allergy completely abated and I remained in Guadalajara for the remainder of my planned two-month stay.

If you think this tall tale of my sensational recovery is just too much, too cut-and-dried, I can empathize with you. I have told you that I also dislike tall tales and also promised you that I would refrain from any form of exaggeration. And I tell you now that the story I told you is true. The only reason I'm pushing this point is that I'm trying to impress on you the value of deep breathing. I only hope my experience was typical and that others may be able to obtain the same degree of relief provided they put in the effort. As for me, I plan to keep breathing exercise a permanent part of my health regime. What inspires me in part to do this is that now I so often experience that deeply satisfying and gratifying feeling that comes with a good, deep lungful of air.

Important caution: Your effort to expand should be just strong enough for you to feel a little tension in the structures of your rib cage, before you begin to feel any real pain. A few light "clicking" sounds should be welcome, as they signify that you are breaking out of stagnation, or the "set," of the structures in this area, gradually building up the size and flexibility of your rib cage and lungs. Notice that I mentioned "your effort to expand..." I did not say to hold your breath by locking your throat. Doing so to hold in a lungful of pressurized air is dangerous and at best puts a strain on your blood vessels, especially those of your eyes. Some years ago a well known bodybuilder was rendered all but blind purportedly from this practice. He ended up wearing very thick eyeglasses and voiced strong regret for having ever trained with weights.

Just one more thing I want to say about the bed exercises: In addition to enjoying them the rest of your life, you would do well to do similar exercises in the course of your usual day, modifying and adapting them as required to suit your situation. As you grow older, especially valuable will be the moves that will minimize your getting "stooped"; namely, those that bend you backward. Push your pelvic and abdominal areas forward, bend your back and head backward and extend your hands behind you. Simultaneously do a little twisting. Pull your shoulders back and try to bring the blades together. Try to touch your shoulders to your ears, both simultaneously at first, then individually. Develop a feel for what is happening to your joints and tissues. Also maintaining a childlike spirit will help you retain your youth longer.

I have told you how I limber up my body and exercise my lungs. You may want to emulate me or innovate your own methods. However you do them, do them. Once a day is good; several times would be better. Within reason it's hard to get too much but easy to not get enough.

Walking, running, and weight training are common and popular enough to have inspired abundant literature on them, and so I will not devote much book space to them.

Instead let us devote more attention to more offbeat, though very beneficial, activities. But I must say that, all things considered, walking must rate as one of the very best exercises of all. It's easy and pleasant, requires no special equipment, can be social, and can be aerobic to whatever degree you want it to be.

REBOUNDING. Rebounding is bouncing on a rebounder, which is simply a small trampoline, downsized to be used mostly in the home for simple health-purposed exercise. A typical rebounder, sometimes informally called a bouncer, would be about 38" in diameter and 9" high. It consists of a durable web of plastic fabric stretched tight across a strong metal ring supported by six short legs. Coil springs provide the bounce. While we're discussing the physical equipment I may as well say that a suitable rebounder can be bought at some discount stores for not much more than $20, making it a real bargain relative to the benefits it offers. I saw one of fair quality recently at a discount store for $10.95, an even better bargain.

Be informed: If you are one of those souls who insist on nothing but the best, you can find some rebounders to accommodate your fine tastes at close to $200 and sometimes more than that. Some of them come with attached hand rails for stability and safety. Only the feeble or unsteady should need these rails.

The rebounder is not designed for the acrobatics performed on a trampoline. Though fancy moves are possible on it, the simple act of bouncing up and down already constitutes the major part of the benefits available from it. Any other moves would be of secondary value. The simplicity of basic rebounding belies the benefits it provides. Contrary to the common opinion, aerobics, while possible and useful on a rebounder, are not nearly the major consideration.

This is how rebounding enhances health:

Your lymphatic system, a network of vessels considerably more extensive that your blood system, is a very critical component of your immune system. Its basic responsibility is to keep your cells healthy by circulating certain body fluids. It does this by carrying them around in the lymph, a viscous clear fluid which is the main vehicle of the system. But it does not have a circulating pump as does your blood system. For circulating it depends on other body functions, including breathing, but mostly muscle action and moving about of the whole body. A stationary body produces very little circulation, if any, and should not remain motionless for periods longer than required for sufficient rest. This is why a sedentary lifestyle is so inimical to health and why bedridden patients suffer rapid deterioration of their bodies. It is also why "couch potatoes" take upon themselves a certain well deserved stigma. The affectionate and humorous connotation of the name does little to exonerate the slothful ones or minimize the deleterious effects of their action, or lack of action.

Lymph, like blood, moves in only one direction, in effect as though it were governed by one-way valves. So, repeated body motions featured by abrupt changes of direction, are very effective in moving the lymph along in its vessels. A rebounder in use is a lymph-circulating machine. And so important is the circulating of lymph that one doctor has said that with a well circulating lymphatic system it is almost impossible to be sick. This may be an exaggeration but it does make a point.

Now, just how do we rebound? Simply by stepping up onto the mat, or web, of the rebounder and bouncing up and down, gently at first to warm up and then higher a bit later. In fact you may even bounce without leaving the mat. For the purpose of lymph circulation the amplitude of the bounce is not of critical importance. This is another great virtue of rebounding; the elderly and feeble can do it with comparative confidence and safety.

Inasmuch as rebounding will completely circulate the system in a few minutes, it is redundant to bounce for long periods. In other words, much longer is not much better. So the recommended strategy is to bounce often for short periods. Three times a day at five or ten minutes each is much more beneficial that a one-hour session.

Can we use the rebounder for aerobics? Yes, of course. You may bounce as you wish consistent with prudence. If aerobics is one of your aims, the rebounder will accommodate you, not only as well as the road, but in at least three ways more safely. Avoidance of automobile injuries and exhaust fumes are two. To runners whose feet and knees are vulnerable to the impact of paved surfaces but who have a strong need or desire for aerobic activity the gentle bounce of the rebounder can be a very welcome substitute.

So effective is directional change in circulating the lymphatic system that reportedly patients with gangrene who were unable to stand regained their ability to walk by placing their feet on a rebounder while in a wheelchair and while someone else did the bouncing for them. The renewed circulation of the lymph in their feet and legs also renewed the health of those members. Also reportedly, eyes have been dramatically strengthened by the exercise imposed on them by the repeated changes of direction.

Albert Carter, long-time exponent and advocate of trampolining and rebounding, tells some impressive stories of almost unbelievable benefits bestowed on the body by rebounding. He states that he has never lifted weights and yet at the age of 39 could do more than 100 successive one-arm push-ups. His two children, ages 8 and 12 at the time, accompanied their parents on trampoline promotions and regularly participated in the demonstrations, as well as trampolining at home. They did 429 and 479 consecutive sit-ups, stopping only because they had to stop some time.

Aside from requiring equipment to bounce on, rebounding shares several advantages with walking: It rates high on the scale of beneficiality, it's not strenuous or expensive, it's comparatively safe, it needs no elaborate or time-consuming gearing-up beforehand nor ungearing after. Rebounding, moreover, can and should be done barefooted, thus saving the costs of special shoes. Perhaps you're beginning to understand why rebounding has often been called the best exercise of all. Perhaps you would like to try it out for yourself. For twenty bucks you can hardly go wrong.

REFLEXOLOGY. While reflexology is not truly exercise, let's discuss it here anyway. It is also known by several other names, though not always accurately; e.g., zone therapy, reflex therapy, reflex massage, shiatsu, acupressure. Though I'm convinced by experience of the validity of this form of therapy, I find it a bit difficult to get all excited over specific remedies for symptom relief. To me they are good adjuncts to the more generalized systemic therapies but no more. There's nothing wrong with them, just so they're not relied on as a cure and no harmful substances are imposed on the patient. Reflexology falls into this class of specific remedy, as do its affiliated practices, acupuncture included. Anyway, dispose of someone's painful symptom and he's happy for it. So who am I to discount the benefits of this practice. And comfort is part of happiness, and after all isn't happiness what we're striving for? Whatever the characteristics of reflexology are, they're all positive, even when the therapist makes you jump in temporary pain.

Reflexology is an art, or technique — not yet a science — of symptom relief by means of pressure applied to certain areas of the body, most popularly the feet, which are intimately connected, or related, to the parts of the body suffering the symptoms.

This form of massage supposedly has been practiced in China for more than 50 centuries. Certain aspects of it are shared with acupuncture, though needles are not used.

The bridge between the suffering part and its pressure point is a component of the nervous system commonly referred to as a meridian, or a channel of energy. Specialists in this field have divided the body into ten longitudinal meridians, and every body part falls into one of these ten.

Reflexology nurtures the thesis that crystalline deposits, mostly uric acid, form at the nerve endings, most of them in the feet and hands. The stagnation which encourages the formation of these crystals may be caused by any of several conditions; e.g., poor circulation, defective associated body part, lack of stimulation of the nerve endings due to the wearing of shoes. The cause-and-effect relationship between a body part and its related crystalline deposit seems to be mutual; i.e., either may be the cause and together they maintain a vicious circle until one of them is remedied. Disintegration and dissipation of the crystal from the reflex point removes the "short circuit" and supposedly restores health to the part by restoring normalcy to its nerve function.

Removal of the crystal is accomplished with massage of the reflex area. Enough pressure is applied to crush the crystal, which is not very hard. But don't try to convince the patient of the softness of the crystal, because when one is pressed, sharp pain is usually experienced, often causing the therapist to be accused of sticking the patient with his or her thumbnail. It's usually "her," because where there is pain a woman is usually involved. The correct area to be pressed is sometimes indicated by the response of the patient to the pressure. When the patient says, "Ouch!," it is determined that a crystal is there, and the therapist will work to dispose of it. However, an experienced therapist will often know the right locations just by listening to the patient's complaints of his or her symptoms. It's usually "his," because men are the weaker sex. In addition to freeing the meridian of the stifling object, the pressure acts as a stimulus activating an electrochemical nerve impulse which restores normal conditions to the body part.

Some crystals require more than one massage session to eradicate, as practitioners are reluctant to effect physiological changes too rapidly lest a too-severe cleansing reaction occur and subject the patient to excessively unpleasant symptoms.

Reflex massage may concentrate on relief of specific symptoms or it may endeavor to enhance all body functions by massaging all reflex locations, which in the foot aspect of reflexology would be the whole of both feet. The hands also contain reflex areas of nerve endings. In disciplines like shiatsu, reflex points exist in numerous places over the body, including the head.

Working on one's own feet is understandably difficult, and so unless one is extraordinarily dedicate to exploring this beneficial technique he must seek the help of others, either a professional or a personal friend. A friend or spouse similarly dedicated would be a great asset.

Let me say before leaving this subject that in addition to being an ancient art in the Orient, in more recent times reflexology has been studied and practiced in many countries of the Western world, and its validity is being increasingly confirmed even among Establishment physicians, who no doubt are frowned upon by their peers and their governing body for their wayward practice.

TAI CHI. (Tai: big, great. Chi: spirit, life force). Tai Chi, an ancient Chinese set of exercises for health, entails slow and graceful movements which purportedly enhance the health of body and mind. Its merits seem to be borne out by its immense popularity, still growing ten centuries after its origination. In Kowloon's Tam Sham Shui Park I went for an early morning stroll about 6 a.m. and was amazed to see several hundreds of people doing Tai Chi, most of them older people, some very old, obviously in it for health rather than the body beautiful. In Tiananmein Square in Beijing I encountered the same spectacle about the same time of day. The huge number of exercisers, their advanced ages, their fervor, convinced me of the efficacy of Tai Chi, or at least its popularity.

Let me excerpt from "Health Benefits of Tai Chi," an article by Ann Sutherland, B.S.C., physical therapist:

"...it is a complete and integrated exercise, one which works all the body's systems deeply yet gently. This makes it an exercise suitable for persons of all ages and conditions for health. ...works muscles, joints, tendons, and ligaments throughout the body, gently stretching them and relaxing them. ...also improves the functions of other physiological systems by increasing the circulation of blood and oxygen to all parts of the body. ...Tai Chi has been found to reduce high blood pressure. ...can reduce the natural degeneration of the spine and/or joints that occur with age. All these effects combine to make Tai Chi a means of

reducing and preventing stress-related diseases. Learning Tai Chi is learning to relax."

I must tell you that Tai Chi, as beneficial as it's purported to be, can try your patience. It is slow and not at all dynamic. If you're a professional fighter or a football player you'd be tempted to walk out of the room at the start of a Tai Chi demonstration. And yet, paradoxically, you would be one who could benefit from this discipline more than most. After mastering the "standard" set of movements — of which there are 108 — the devotee could venture into advanced degrees of training which take him into the martial arts. I have been told that the movements here are "lightning-fast" and a far cry from the super-slow basic movements, and that the masters of this art are extraordinarily formidable fighters. Not that I want you to be a fighter; be a lover.

An almost infinite number and variety of exercises are available for health. We have discussed just a few of them. If you're inclined, investigate on your own and select activities that meet your criteria for promotion of health while being enjoyable enough to inspire you to carry through on your program. You might enjoy punching the speed bag, jumping rope, water exercises, aerobic classes, television exercise shows, or whatever suits your fancy. I have purposely refrained from discussing jogging and running. Jogging is commonplace and adequately covered by other writers. Running, like some other competitive sports, generally goes beyond the degree of effort required for health purposes. If you enjoy the effects of running, fine, but it is not my idea of a preferred health exercise.

Again, include your mind and spirit in all that you do for your health. They are your board of directors and your cheering section.

REST

Rest is not "just" rest. It is not just doing nothing. It isn't just the cessation of the expenditure of energy. Nor does the replenishment of energy cap off the definition of rest. Somewhat as the volume of the autonomic functions of your brain outweigh its conscious thoughts, the less obvious functions of rest are far more extensive than we generally realize. So if you make a lifestyle of overwork, overplay, under- or over-rest, careless dietary habits, and neglect of your spirit, you will tend to have a less-than-ideal old age, if you live long enough to be old.

Rest is a nourishing as well as a cleansing process. Besides the preservation and replenishment of energy, a very considerable, in fact essential, benefit of rest is the restoration of homeostasis, a state of physiological equilibrium produced by a balance of functions and chemical composition. Homeostasis is not as readily recognized nor as directly felt as are the other benefits, though it is at the very core of health. For this reason many people fail to allow enough rest time for the body to accomplish its mission. As soon as they feel a return of energy, or even only a relief from exhaustion, they begin to again subject their bodies to stresses. Though this attitude is sometimes admirable, especially when the activity resumed or initiated is wholesome and productive, it accelerates the aging process. So it is a good practice to rest not only until fatigue mitigates but if convenient for some time after. A moderate amount of laziness is not altogether a bad thing. As Socrates said, be moderate in all things. Please realize that you're not necessarily a hero when you overwork. Insufficient rest deprives the body of time to restore homeostasis. Too much rest allows stagnation of and jeopardy to the whole body, including the immune system.

What is sleep? Does the lack of consciousness featured by sleep afford us any benefits not available from waking rest? Yes, it does. Sleep is rest for the brain, the conscious mind, and the other nerves. When you're awake, even though sitting or lying motionless, it is almost impossible to keep your brain and other nerves from working, and so they fail to rest and fail to regenerate. This is why serious insomniacs are generally less than happy and not quite up to snuff. And of course unhealthy and unhappy people don't sleep well either; and so it's a vicious circle. And the best way I know to short out the circle is to commit yourself to a healthy lifestyle.

A healthy body requires less sleep, because it houses a healthier, more durable, brain and nervous system which can run longer before requiring regeneration. This is not to say that sleep regenerates only the brain and other nerves, because, as we know, our bodies and spirits respond happily to a good restful sleep. And remember, we have said repeatedly that the entire body is a well orchestrated integration of interdependent and interacting parts.

There is no shortage of literature on sleep, but let me submit a few comments:

1. Healthy bodies, including brains and minds, sleep better.

2. Being healthy includes being well nourished. The B vitamins are known to enhance the health of the brains and other nerves, which promote mental tranquillity and restful sleep. Two popular natural sources of the B vitamins are brewer's yeast and desiccated liver.

3. People who exercise, both physically and mentally, sleep better. "Couch potatoes" tend to sleep poorly. And what sleep they do get cannot as effectively help a body which refuses to participate in a wholesome lifestyle.

Any way we can alleviate the regenerative task of our

bodies will facilitate the whole project and tend to enhance our health. One effective measure we can exploit to this end is fasting, a rest for the digestive system. It is not for nothing that fasting is mentioned so often in written history. It indeed is a great boon to our bodies. America is overfed and undernourished. Relieved of its digestive duties by a fast, the body can more effectively fulfill its other functions, such as restoration of energy and purgation of toxins. It should be obvious that cleansing can never be completed while food, especially junk, is being stuffed into the body. So fasting now and then has been employed by many people throughout the world and throughout history as a means of purging impurities and rejuvenating health. And while not fasting we can help the cause by minimizing the consumption of junk food.

Fasting and rest are discussed also in the chapter on Internal Cleanliness.

I hope we can see that rest benefits us in major, though inconspicuous, ways and that we should appreciate and utilize it accordingly. While the use-it-or-lose-it concept is valid as concerns our energy supply, it is also true that the replenishment of a used resource will prolong the supply of the resource. It is also true that the efficiency of physiological functions are jeopardized by the presence of chemical and physical trash and enhanced by a clean environment fee of foreign and interfering influences. Rest aims to enhance this efficiency.

SUMMARY

1. Minimize the quantities of free radicals, because these are the gremlins that attack all the cells of our bodies and age us before our time.
2. Optimize the quality and quantities of antioxidants,

because these are the substances that render the free radicals harmless by neutralizing their effects. Provide adequate amounts of quality building materials to enhance and maintain a healthy body.

3. Maintain a wholesome mind and spirit, because we know that our entire being is made up of the body, the mind, and the spirit, and that the health of one intimately affects the others.

4. Exercise the body also, in order to maintain a healthy tone of our entire physiology, which in turn will enhance mental and spiritual health.

5. Allow adequate rest for your body and mind. Physical rest allows the body to cleanse and nourish itself with the wholesome food we eat. Sleep is rest for the mind and spirit.

I hope I have given you useful material to contemplate. But in contemplating, do not entertain the attitude that you're going to try out the concepts and recommendations I have offered you. They may not be perfect but are based on truth and love and are the best approach I have found. And after all, what other choices do we have? Big Medi$in? It has its place but doesn't fill the bill. When you come down to it, it is you who is on trial. It is your health and your money. You pass the test and Mother will do the rest.

I am not going to wish you luck, because luck isn't going to do it. But I do wish you the wisdom to appreciate the worthwhileness of being a responsible steward of the temple of the Holy Spirit, and the strength of resolve to fulfill that responsibility. I also wish you a long life of glowing health and happiness, because God loves you and so do I.

APPENDIX

READING I HAVE LIKED

Abundant good literature not only on true health but also on the abundant untrue health practices is available in libraries, book stores, and health stores. Monthly health advisory letters, mostly by enlightened researchers, await your subscription. Many of them are well worth their price, some around $39 per year.

To be sure, not every printed word on the subject is true blue, but as my favorite teacher used to teach us, "Some books are to be tasted, others to be swallowed, and some few to be chewed and digested."

The list below represents only a small portion of what has been written on the subject. Some of the books are old and out of print, and some others are minor and inconspicuous works that hardly excited the health and literary communities. But I liked them and choose to list them here on the chance that they will somehow show up in your sphere.

Death by Prescription — William A. Siler
Doctors on Trial — John H. Bradshaw, M.D.
Medical Wars — Roger Pirnie Doyle
Medical Care Costs — Barrett
The Doctor Disagrees — Elizabeth Seifert
The Doctor's Confession — Elizabeth Seifert
The Doctor's Kingdom — Elizabeth Seifert
Doctor on Trial — Elizabeth Seifert
The Plague Makers — Jeffrey A. Fisher, M.D.
The Doctor Game — Howard Olgin

The Doctor Business — (Author Unknown)
Dr. Sam, an American Tragedy — Jack Harrison Pollock
Medical Ethics — Colen, BD
Medical Ethics — Heintze
Medical Ethics — Maklin
Medical Ethics — Weir
Medical Ethics — Weiss
Racketeering in Medicine, the Suppression of Alternatives
    — James P. Carter, M.D.
Is Hearth Surgery Necessary? — Julian Whitaker, M.D.
Health and Healing — Andrew Weil, M.D.
Chiropractic Speaks Out — Chester A. Wilk, M.D.
The Challenge and Effort of Traditional Medicine
    — Julius H. Tsuei
What Your Doctor Didn't Learn in Medical School
    — Stuart M. Berger
Sweet and Dangerous — John Yudkin, M.D.
Sugar Blues — William Duffy
Body, Mind and Sugar — E.M. Abrahamson, M.D.,
    and A.W. Pezet
Hypoglycemia and You — Carlton Fredericks, M.D.
Hypoglycemia: A Better Approach — Paavo Airola, N.D.
Fresh Food versus Stale Food — Robert Ford
How Nature Cures — Emmet Densmore, M.D.
Healing for the Age of Enlightenment
    — Stanley Burroughs
The Practical Encyclopedia of Healing — Mark Briklin
Health Secrets From Europe — Paavo Airola, N.D.
Are You Confused? — Paavo Airola, N.D.
There IS a Cure for Arthritis — Paavo Airola, N.D.
A Cancer Therapy - Fifty Cases — Max Gerson, M.D.
The Cancer Answer — Maureen Salaman

Censured For Curing Cancer — S.J. Haught
The Cancer Cure That Worked — Barry Lynes
Inner Cleansing — Carlson Wade
Nine-Day Inner Cleansing and Blood Wash for Renewed
   Youthfulness and Health
   — I.E. Gaumont and Harold E. Buttram, M.D.
Dr. Wright's Book of Nutritional Therapy
   — Jonathan V. Wright, M.D.
The Fountain of Youth — C.E. Butis
The Milk of Human Kindness is Not Pasteurized
   — William Douglass Campbell, M.D.
Diet for a Small Planet — Frances Moore Lappe
You Mean I'm Not Lazy, Crazy, or Stupid?
   — Kate Kelly & Peggy Ramundo
Mental Health Through Nutrition — Tom R. Blaine
Psycho-Nutrition — Carlton Fredericks, M.D.
There's a Lot More to Health Than Not Being Sick
   — Bruce Larson, Ph.D.
The Book of Health — Susan Stockton
Nutrition for Health — Alice Chase, D.O.
Silent Spring — Rachel Carson
Hunza Health Secrets — Renee Taylor
Secret to Hunza Superior Health — Carl Classic
Free Radicals — Zane Baranowski
Health Freedom News — P.O. Box 688, Monrovia,
   CA 91017 (818) 357-2181
Prevention (Magazine) — Emmaus, PA 18049
Let's Live (Magazine) — P.O. Box 74908, Los Angeles,
   CA 90004-3030
Health Sciences Institute Monthly Newsletter
   — 105 W. Monument St., Baltimore, MD 21201
   (410) 223-2611

BOOKS THAT CAN TRANSFORM LIVES

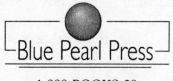